W9-AAK-376

GLEN C. CAIN

LONG

THE ECONOMICS OF
HEALTH

THE ECONOMICS OF

HEALTH

HERBERT E. KLARMAN

COLUMBIA UNIVERSITY PRESS

New York and London, 1965

Copyright © 1965 Columbia University Press
Library of Congress Catalog Card Number: 65-14323
Manufactured in the United States of America

FOREWORD

This monograph is one of a series of three dealing with the economics of health, education, and welfare. In commissioning these volumes, the Ford Foundation was influenced by the fact that expenditures in these three fields are in excess of $100 billion annually, that they are among the most important and sensitive areas of the entire economy, and that communication between economists and those making policy and operating decisions in these areas has been infrequent and irregular.

Of the three areas, health economics is perhaps the most neglected by economists, and it is hoped that this volume will serve a dual purpose of interesting not only medical personnel, hospital administrators, and legislators charged with determining the amount and direction of flow of public funds to health, but also economists. Dr. Herbert E. Klarman has had a long-standing interest in the economics of health and has been a leading contributor to the literature in this area. Therefore, he was a logical choice to undertake a review of past work and to suggest future research opportunities. Professor Klarman's colleagues will appreciate his succinct and knowledgeable review of the literature and may find themselves stimulated to make their own research contributions to this vital area of public policy.

The other two monographs in the series are *The Economic Value of Education*, by Professor T. W. Schultz of the University of Chicago, and *The Economics of Welfare Policies*, by Dr. Margaret S. Gordon of the University of California (Berkeley). All three authors have been free to develop and interpret the materials in their chosen field according to their own judgment; the views expressed are, of course, their own. The Ford Foundation is grateful to them for the time and care that they have devoted to this important task.

Marshall A. Robinson, *Director*
Program in Economic Development
and Administration

New York City
July, 1964

ACKNOWLEDGMENTS

The author is grateful to the following colleagues and friends for reading the manuscript of this book and offering comments and criticisms:

Carl F. Christ, Department of Political Economy, The Johns Hopkins University

Peter E. de Janosi, Ford Foundation

Rashi Fein, Brookings Institution

Victor R. Fuchs, formerly with the Ford Foundation and now with the National Bureau of Economic Research

Richard Goode, Brookings Institution

Dale Hiestand, Graduate School of Business, Columbia University

Edwin S. Mills, Department of Political Economy, The Johns Hopkins University

Mary A. Monk, School of Hygiene and Public Health, The Johns Hopkins University

Charles M. Wylie, School of Hygiene and Public Health, The Johns Hopkins University

It goes without saying that responsibility for errors (of commission and omission) remains with the undersigned.

The manuscript was typed and retyped a number of times. Miss Selma Cohen did this herself or closely supervised the work of others. Jules Altman prepared the index.

Baltimore   Herbert E. Klarman
May 28, 1964

CONTENTS

I. OVERVIEW

The availability and the financing of health and medical services of good quality preoccupy large numbers of the American people some of the time and some people almost all of the time. Among the latter is the small group of so-called health economists, that is, persons who work on problems of financing, pricing, staffing, and organizing health and medical services in this country.

A major objective of this monograph is to engage the interest of economists in the problems of the health field, with the hope that more of them may wish to spend time working on these problems. The objective is approached along several routes: by reviewing the work that economists have performed in health and medical care; by relating this work to the mainstream of economic literature; and by indicating some of the interesting and important questions that await exploration. At the same time this book is intended to acquaint the intelligent lay public and professional health personnel with the approaches, analytical methods, and viewpoints that economists bring to the health field and to convey in plain (but not simple) English the substantive contributions of economics to this field.

The opening chapter comprises three sections: (*a*) an attempt to define the economics of health; (*b*) a short description of the health and medical care industry; and (*c*) a delineation of the distinctive economic characteristics of health and medical services.

A. WHAT IS THE ECONOMICS OF HEALTH?

Conceptually the economics of health is the application of economics to the health field. This definition is not very revealing, since health services fall outside the traditional preoccupations of applied economics. It is helpful at the outset to examine what health economics is generally considered to be and how economists regard their contribution to the health field. Most medical schools offer lectures in medical economics. These cover a wide range of subjects—from advice on the location, organization, and businesslike operation of a practitioner's office through a description of the health and medical care industry, usually in numerical terms, to a discussion of the politics of compulsory health insurance [24, p. 786]. Most often medical economics is taken to deal with money or financial questions in the field of health or with the financing of medical care, medical education, and medical research.

Often lacking in such lectures and in the published literature of the medical professions and hospitals is the view of economics as a way of thinking about and approaching issues of public policy in financing and organizing health and medical services [63, p. 5]. Rarely encountered is the notion that economics is a toolbox for analyzing problems [33, p. 1].

The economics of health is a newer term than medical economics. It is a broader term that proposes to encompass the medical care industry, as the former term did, and also to extend beyond it into such fields as the analysis of the economic costs of diseases and the benefits of control programs, returns from investment in education and training, the conditions conducive to medical research, and so forth.

In a formal sense the economics of health may be defined as the economic aspects of health services—those aspects of the health problem that deal with the determination of the quantity and prices of the scarce resources devoted to this and related purposes and with the combinations in which these resources are employed. Since the economic problem must be solved for a specific form of social organization or institutional framework [11, p. 7], the discussion and analysis of the economic aspects of health must pertain to the choices facing a given country or locality with its particular resources, forms of organization, and methods of payment. Typically, the economist's contribution is to state the costs (or, what is the same, the consequences in terms of opportunities foregone) of alternative courses of action.

In so doing he assumes a measure of responsibility for the quality of the data he handles, asking how accurately they measure what they purport to measure. It is recognized that the distinction between means and ends is not always clear [35, pp. 328-29]. Some economists include within their purview the formulation of goals and priorities for public policy, giving explicit statement to the various considerations involved, including their own value judgments [37, p. 62].

Greenfield includes within the scope of health economics the population problem; the quantity and quality of resources allocated to the health area; the medical care industry's efficiency; losses due to illness, disability, and premature death; possible economies of scale (lower costs associated with increased volume of services); and relationships between the organization and financing of the industry and its function [14, p. 4].

For the sake of concreteness, if not for reasons of space, it is necessary to limit the scope of inquiry. It is accepted that a people's health is influenced by heredity and by such factors in their environment and standard of living as food, housing, sanitation, and education [12, p. 734; 19, p. 18; 55, p. 941; 65, p. 143]. Indeed, it is claimed that medical care made little or no contribution to the health of its recipients before the nineteenth century [20, p. 141]. "The conquest of epidemic disease was in large part the result of the campaign for pure food, pure water, and pure air based not on scientific doctrine but on philosophical faith" [8, p. 125]. While the capacity of medical care to contribute to health and life expectancy has vastly increased in the twentieth century, the important contribution of the other factors continues to be recognized.

Although not central to the argument, some comments on what is meant by health may be in order. Today the popular definition of health derives from the Preamble to the Constitution of the World Health Organization: "Health means more than freedom from disease, freedom from pain, freedom from untimely death. It means optimum physical, mental, and social efficiency and well-being." This definition is probably too broad to furnish guidance regarding a society's real aims in the health field and too vague for the purpose of evaluating existing programs. Moreover, mental and social states are difficult to define. It is also doubtful that most individuals or societies pursue health with single-minded devotion. H. L. Mencken wrote: "One of the chief objects of medicine is to save us from the natural consequences of our vices and follies." The stated goal may be too static, insofar as health may be regarded as a process of continuing adaptation [8, p. 233].

From a practical point of view, it makes sense to focus on the health and medical care industry as it is defined by the authorities who produce the data on finances and manpower. How is this industry staffed, equipped, organized, and financed?

B. THE HEALTH AND MEDICAL CARE INDUSTRY

A detailed description of the health and medical care industry is given by Somers and Somers [42]. Here selected data are presented together with a brief text. Sources of data are cited, and the quality of data is appraised.

Personnel, Facilities, and Organization
As of 1960, it is estimated, the health and medical care industry employed between 2.5 and 3.0 million persons, depending on the inclusiveness of the definition employed. The practicing physicians (242,000 plus 14,000 osteopaths) and dentists (101,000), whose professional judgment guides the consumer in the use of health and medical services, comprise 12 to 14 percent of all health manpower [47, p. 28; also letter from Maryland Y. Pennell, U. S. Public Health Service, October 18, 1961]. Altogether, the industry employs persons in some thirty professional and technically skilled categories, in addition to the large numbers of unskilled workers [25, p. 6].

Although some physicians are employed by government, insurance companies, medical schools, and hospitals, the large majority are in private practice. Among the latter most are strictly in solo practice or have some arrangement to share expenses with other physicians.

Physicians employed by the government and other organizations work for a salary, though some hospital physicians have other contractual arrangements, such as a sharing of gross receipts. Self-employed physicians are usually paid on a fee-for-service basis. Capitation payments (a stated periodic amount per enrollee) have been tried in prepaid group practice and in behalf of public charges.

In the past two generations an increasing number and proportion of physicians have come to specialize. The focus of physicians' activities has shifted from patients' homes to physicians' offices and, more recently, to hospitals with their large numbers of nurses, technicians, and auxiliary helpers. Telephone conversations between patients and physicians have attained such magnitude as to be counted as visits by the National Health Survey [42, p. 48].

A higher proportion of dentists than of physicians are in private practice. Relatively few dentists are specialists or work in hospitals [46, pp. 40–43]. Dentists employ a higher ratio of office assistants than do physicians. Almost all of dental care is rendered on a fee-for-service basis and paid for by patients out of pocket, without reimbursement by insurance.

In nursing the major change in the past two generations is the relative shift from private duty nursing to salaried employment, mostly in hospitals. Although a declining proportion of the total, the number of private duty nurses remains high at 70,000. They are private contractors, but most of them work in hospitals where their fees are often subject to approval. Other professional nurses work in doctors' offices, industrial plants, voluntary agencies, public health departments, and schools. Apart from public health nursing and teaching in schools of nursing, there is little specialization. Among the important recent changes in organization are team nursing and assumption by the professional nurse of the role of team leader or manager. Both changes are associated with the postwar increase in the number of married nurses who work part-time and with a huge expansion in auxiliary nursing personnel. In 1960 there were 225,000 practical nurses and 400,000 aides, attendants, and orderlies, in addition to 504,000 registered (professional) nurses [47, p. 28].

Some of the 120,000 pharmacists are employed by hospitals, and some are employed as manufacturers' and wholesalers' rep-

resentatives (detail men), but nearly 90 percent work in retail
pharmacies as owners or employees. The modern retail pharmacist
is not a manufacturer of drugs but a dispenser who is situated in
close proximity to the patient and can fill a prescription on short
notice. All drug stores carry proprietary drugs, as well as prescription drugs, and most carry a large variety of other products.
Prostheses and braces are, however, custom-made and sold
through separate, independent stores.

Drugs are manufactured by pharmaceutical houses or branches
of large chemical firms. The market for a specific drug is characterized by intense competition among a few sellers through
large expenditures on advertising and research and by market
"imperfections," such as emphasis on trade names over generic
names and other efforts to maintain price [25, p. 7]. There is a
high rate of obsolescence of products, owing to scientific advances, continual efforts to overcome the propensity of disease
organisms to acquire resistance to drugs, and competition for the
consumer's dollar.

Of the 1.7 million beds in hospitals in this country, one
tenth are operated by the federal government for its special
charges, two fifths are in short-term hospitals under other ownership, and one half are in long-term hospitals, including mental
and tuberculosis hospitals. Federal hospitals care for the military,
some of their dependents, veterans to varying degrees, and
sailors. Eighty-five percent of the long-term hospital beds are
for patients with mental illness, and these are owned mostly by
the states. Tuberculosis care is predominantly a governmental
function. In short-term hospital care, however, state and local
governments account for only 25 percent of the beds and 20 percent of the admissions. By contrast, voluntary (nonprofit) hospitals own 70 percent of the beds and admit almost three fourths
of the patients. Proprietary (profit) hospitals have 5 percent of
the beds in the nation and admit 6 to 7 percent of the patients
[105, p. 414]. Proprietary hospitals are almost nonexistent in
some parts of the country, but their number is increasing rapidly
in a few metropolitan areas with rapid growth of population, including Los Angeles and suburban New York. Proprietary owners

operate, however, 70 percent of the 362,000 skilled nursing-home beds in the nation [48].

The figures on numbers of physicians and dentists are meant to be complete. These are licensed occupations that a member seldom leaves, so that the professional directory should yield an accurate count [139, pp. 222, 224]. The directory, however, may present some overstatement of active manpower, owing to the inclusion of retired and semiactive practitioners. Sometimes there is an understatement of the number of physicians in the American Medical Association's Directory, owing to a lag in the inclusion of one or two graduating classes and the exclusion of foreign exchange visitors on temporary visas [49; 174, pp. 145–46, 161]. The latter, however, are included in the counts of hospital house staff (interns and residents), so that a discrepancy exists in the data on hospital physicians from these two sources. The figures on nursing personnel formerly grouped students with graduates, underestimated registered nurses in hospitals, and often disregarded auxiliary personnel. These deficiencies have been overcome. There is now an increasing tendency to report data for the other professional health personnel—osteopaths, veterinarians, chiropodists, and so forth. For technicians and less skilled personnel the most reliable counts are for hospital workers.

Similarly, data on facilities and their use are most complete for hospitals [105, pp. 403–50]. Figures on nursing homes and infirmaries in homes for the aged have been collected for a shorter period under the aegis of the state agencies that administer the federal (Hill-Burton) program of grants-in-aid for the construction of nonprofit hospitals. However, the bed figures reported for hospitals and related facilities are those submitted by the institutions and often do not reflect any uniform criteria for measurement. The data on hospital use collected annually by the American Hospital Association are better for inpatients than for outpatients. Data on services in hospitals to private ambulatory patients are poor. The National Health Survey collects data from households on hospital admissions and duration of stay, and is the only source of routine data on the volume of physicians' and dentists' services. There are no readily available data on facilities and equipment outside institutions—in doctors' offices or group practice units.

Expenditures and Sources of Income

Expenditures for health and medical care rose from $3.6 billion in 1929 to $33.8 billion in 1963 [76, Table 1], a more than ninefold increase in thirty-four years, or an average (geometric mean) increase of 6.8 percent a year. When allowance is made for the rise in medical care prices of 227 percent, the rise in real expenditures (in constant dollars) was fourfold.

What do the billions of dollars represent? They include expenditures for health and medical services provided by physicians, hospitals, dentists, nurses, and other health personnel; commodities such as drugs, prosthetic appliances, and medical supplies; public health programs; medical research; part of the costs of training health personnel (principally in hospitals); and a large part of the capital expenditures for physical plant and facilities in the health and medical care industry (mostly hospitals, nursing homes, and health centers) [219, p. 796].

Excluded from the data are expenditures for medical education outside hospitals and the value of contributed services of part-time volunteers in hospitals, including those of physicians. Also excluded are certain items that may have a direct effect on health but fall outside the boundaries of the health and medical care industry—such as expenditures for food, water, housing, education, and recreation—and such items as prescribed diets in the home and transportation to and from physicians' offices and hospitals, the last two being authorized medical expense deductions under the federal individual income tax. Also excluded are economic costs that are not reflected in expenditures for health services and payments that do not entail the use of resources (transfer payments). An example of these economic costs are the so-called indirect costs of disease and injury (loss of output due to disability or premature death). An example of transfer payments are public assistance grants to persons disabled by disease.

Expenditures for health and medical care are frequently related to the value of the economy's output. Two measures of the output of the economy may be used: gross national product (GNP) and net national product (NNP). The former is more widely known and exceeds the latter by the amount of capital consumption (depreciation) in the economy. Between 1929 and 1963 the ratio of health and medical care expenditures to GNP rose from 3.6 to 5.9 percent. During the postwar era it rose by two thirds, climbing slowly in the early 1950s and at a faster pace after 1955. Among the factors making for the large increase in health and medical care expenditures are the rise in prices, which was previously noted, the growth in population, and the higher per capita use of services (attributable, in turn, to advances in medical technology and in the standard of living).

For many years consumer expenditures for health and medical care constituted 4 percent of all consumer expenditures. In the past consumer expenditures for health and medical care were often treated as equivalent to total, or almost total, expenditures, and expenditures by government were disregarded. Since expenditures by business and philanthropy were usually neglected, they were effectively excluded from the total unless they had been incorporated in consumer expenditures.

Even those who sought to go beyond the consumer data and compile a complete figure for health and medical care expenditures sometimes discovered the same constant. Employing United States data for the years 1929 to 1956, Seale found a tendency for health and medical care expenditures to absorb a constant fraction of GNP, that is, 4 percent [38, p. 556].

Today it is known that the true ratio in 1955 was 4.7 percent. However, Seale was working prior to the development of the Social Security Administration (Merriam) series [21], and his figures on health and medical care expenditures were too low. For 1956 Seale's total is $16.3 billion; Merriam's corresponding figure is $19.5 billion ($20.3 billion when expenditures for construction are added). Two billion dollars of the discrepancy are due to an understatement in the data by the National Income Division of the U. S. Department of Commerce, which was subsequently corrected.

Approximately three fifths of the financing of health and medical care comes from consumers, who are assisted by prepayment through insurance plans. Employer contributions to health insurance account for 10 percent [76, Table 3]. Philanthropic contributions play a relatively small role in the over-all picture—3.5 percent—but are of strategic importance in certain hospitals. Government's 24 percent of the total pays for public health services, two thirds of all medical research, and medical care for designated groups in the population.

The data on expenditures by business, philanthropy, government, and health insurance are prepared by the Social Security Administration and published annually in the *Social Security Bulletin* (recently in the November issue). In the figures for private expenditures no distinction is made between health insurance premiums paid by consumers and those paid by employers. The estimate of philanthropy is derived from fragmentary data and appears to lack a firm basis [88, p. 102]. The estimates of government expenditures and health insurance draw on many sources and are believed to be reasonably complete.

The data on consumer expenditures for health and medical care are based essentially on reports from producers. Developed initially by the National Income Division of the Department of Commerce (and published annually in the *Survey of Current Business*, July issue), they are later adjusted by the Social Security Administration (and published in the *Social Security Bulletin*, December issue). Comparison with aggregate data derived from a household survey shows sizable discrepancies in the aggregates for physicians, hospitals, and dentists, after adjustment for differences in definition [75a, Table II]. The figures on expenditures for drugs agree. Yet this was the item that required the largest adjustment—more than $1 billion—when the National Income Division revised its data for the year 1956.

C. DISTINCTIVE ECONOMIC CHARACTERISTICS

Few economists work actively on the problems of the health field. One reason is probably the same as that given by Peterson for sociologists: economists prefer to work on their own problems [178, pp. 2–3]. Another reason is given by health economists. It is Mushkin's belief that economists pay little attention to the health field because the special characteristics of health and medical services mark them as exceptions to the economic propositions that explain the behavior of the market [24, p. 786]. Most economists who have inquired into the provision of health and medical services support this view [1, p. 255; 2, pp. 400–1; 36b, p. 122; 43b, pp. 219–20; 60, p. 290; 229, p. viii], though they may disagree on the policy implications of holding it.

By contrast, Lees believes that health or medical services—he uses the terms interchangeably—have no economic characteristics that differentiate them sharply from other goods [19, pp. 19–21]. The writer agrees that for any single characteristic of health services that is presumably distinctive it may be possible to find an analogue in the behavior of some other good or service. What is rare or unlikely, however, is another good that shares all of these characteristics or so many.

The major distinctive economic characteristics of health and medical services are listed below. Following each is a brief statement that seeks to spell out some of the implications of the distinctions.

Uneven and unpredictable incidence of illness. Apart from periodic physical examinations and immunization procedures that can be scheduled, requirements for health and medical services depend on the incidence of illness and injury. It is possible to predict rates of illness for a population on the basis of past experience. For an individual, illness is not predictable. Although he can try to save money in order to defray the costs of illness, he cannot be sure that he will accumulate a sufficient amount in time. Moreover, illness entails also the risk of impairment or loss of earning ability [55, p. 949].

An obvious implication of the uncertain incidence of illness for an individual and predictable experience for the group is the desirability of pooling payments to meet the contingency of illness in the group. Pooling has taken the form of prepayment, because a service is not repossessable by the seller in the manner of a car or other durable goods. Moreover, the patient may be reluctant or unable to post-pay for services that he received in the dim past and may no longer appreciate. Receipt of care from physicians and hospitals is often associated with pain, discomfort, and personal indignity and is not always recalled with pleasure or satisfaction. In illness such care is not desired but is sought because of the possibly drastic consequences of going without it.

Another distinction arises because some health and medical services occur regularly whereas others are associated with illness, which is unpredictable. The cost of regular, expected services may be prepaid but cannot be insured; the cost of occasional, unexpected services can be both prepaid and insured. Moreover, some types of health and medical service, such as visits to a physician, are regarded as less subject to actuarial control than others, such as admission to a hospital, and are associated with greater "moral hazard." The proper purpose of voluntary health insurance in this country—protection against major risks of illness or injury versus family budgeting of all or most costs of medical care—has been an object of controversy since its inception in the mid-1930s.

External effects. By definition, external effects in economics involve good and bad results for others that flow from one's own behavior [36c, p. 478].

In case of a communicable disease, provision of a preventive or curative service to an individual yields a benefit beyond the prevention or cure of illness in that individual. When a chain of infection is broken, the effect achieved is manyfold that for the person who received the treatment. Moreover, when a sizable proportion of a population has achieved immunity to a disease, the risk of infection for all others is reduced. In such instances, the economist states, the private marginal benefit from an expenditure is less than the social marginal benefit. If so, consumer demand expressed through the market is too low.

As noted below (p. 17), the coupling of service and education is another example of extra buyer benefits that may be associated with the consumption of health and medical services. Medical research is an example of an external economy that can be realized only through public action, since sooner or later the results of research are widely diffused [36c, p. 805].

Health and medical care as a need. A person's need for

health and medical care is generally taken as the basis of his right to receive it, regardless of ability to pay. The medical profession has always acknowledged an obligation to meet this need or an essential part of it. As a consequence, it provides free care to the poor and applies a sliding scale of fees (varying charges in relation to ability to pay) to the population at large. Hospital care, too, is provided at full pay, at part pay, or free, depending on the patient's means.

The right of all sick persons to receive health and medical care according to need represents the expressed consensus of all segments of American society and every shade of political opinion [130, p. 633]. Although a person's income and assets are known to influence the volume of health and medical services he receives and perhaps also their quality (certainly the amenities), we like to believe that nobody goes without the adequate minimum merely because he cannot pay.

Free health and medical care goes beyond the population group on public assistance (relief) and is extended to the "medically indigent" (persons who normally can pay their way but cannot afford to bear the extraordinary costs of illness). Criteria of medical indigence vary widely from community to community and even among government departments and voluntary agencies within the same community. At a given time criteria of eligibility for free care depend on the amount of available funds as well as on an agency's social philosophy and long-range aims [174, p. 408]. In large cities hospitals care, at public expense, for several (four, five, or six) times as many medically indigent persons as indigent ones.

A sliding scale and similar arrangements may succeed in bringing adequate health and medical care to all the people in a community that possesses ample resources of health personnel and facilities. By making possible a higher concentration of physicians in areas with above average income without commensurate loss in physician income, a sliding scale serves, however, to aggravate the unequal geographic distribution of physicians [92, p. 680; 141, p. 11].

Application of a sliding scale presupposes that the physician has knowledge of the patient's ability to pay. In the past, this ability has been measured in terms of the patient's income and assets. The rise of health insurance, which enhances a person's ability to pay for the insured service, complicates matters. If the sliding scale is applied literally, it may offset the value of the health insurance benefit. If so, why should people buy insurance?

Purchasing power to pay for one's wants is not the sole difference between the medical concept of need and the economist's concept of demand. It has been stated that a medical need may exist even when an individual is not aware of it or does not appreciate the potential efficacy of medical care in meeting it [114, p. 324; 134, pp. 11–12]. Owing to its increased effectiveness because of scientific advances, health and medical care is now proposed as the fourth human necessity, ranking after food, clothing, and shelter [15, p. 4; 29, vol. 1, p. 1]. Such a necessity is deemed to have an absolute priority among society's goals.

Among economists it is generally accepted that we cannot afford to do all the things that people need and that would be useful. A particular health program is justified not because it is necessary or good but because it constitutes a better use of resources than some alternative program [10, p. 25].

Lack of knowledge. Another characteristic of health and medical services is the consumer's inability to evaluate them [37, p. 334]. He cannot judge quality even after he has received the services. When the patient says that care is poor, he is often correct; when he says that it is good, he may be mistaken [186, p. 22]. The consumer is incompetent at buying a good that is complex and rarely purchased, such as an appendectomy [43a, p. 66]; he is inexperienced [55, p. 951].

The consumer's inability to judge the quality of health and medical care is not exclusively his. It is associated with an inability on the part of physicians and administrators to observe and measure the specific effects of most services on the health of individuals. Experts, therefore, have come to employ as an index of quality the conditions that surround the provision of care [174, pp. 300–2].

A person chooses a physician but does not himself determine

how much care he will obtain [124, p. 157]. Once the patient
decides to seek help, it is the physician who decides what kind
of services will be rendered and how often, and it is the physician who prescribes the other goods and services, such as drugs
and hospital care, that should supplement or replace his own
services. Needless to say, every patient does not follow his
physician's advice.

The consumer's ignorance and helplessness place a heavy
responsibility on the integrity and the competence of the physician. This is recognized through the Hippocratic oath administered to physicians at graduation from medical school. Licensure by the states constitutes practical recognition of this
fact in modern times [55, pp. 965–66]. Hospitals are subject in
some states to licensure, in other states to more flexible types
of official supervision, and everywhere to voluntary accreditation
and approval of educational programs by professional associ-
ations.

Even state licensure and official regulation tend to be
dominated or controlled by the profession, on the ground that it
alone possesses the requisite expertise. The desire and the
power of an occupational group to promote quality cannot always be dissociated from the opportunity to reduce competition [74, p. 28].

Conditions for effective competition are not favorable in
medicine. On the one hand, the possibility of substituting services afforded by cultists or by persons in professions requiring
less formal training are viewed with disfavor by the community
at large. On the other hand, to insist on expanding the medical
profession in line with some accepted criteria of economic
optima may have the effect of promoting an increase in the volume of prescribed visits [140, p. 8]. The practicability of competition among hospitals is reduced by the high proportion of
fixed costs and by the unique physician-hospital relationship.

Mixture of consumption and investment elements. For the
most part health and medical services are viewed as consumption items. Sometimes seen as necessities, they are also elements of a rising standard of living.

Failure to render medical care to a gainfully occupied member of the labor force who needs it may result in disability and loss of output. Hence, medical benefits, including rehabilitation services, are provided under workmen's compensation.

A program aimed at preventing illness and disability among productive workers is obviously more of an investment in the nation's output than one that extends needed medical services to aged persons who are retired from the labor force. However, humane grounds for providing care are not invalid grounds. They merely fall outside the purview of the special competence of the economist.

Large component of personal service. Most health and medical services are personal services or embody a large component of personal service [25, p. 6]. This fact has important implications for an economy that grows mainly through gains in productivity, rather than through expansion of the labor force. Thus, hospitals, which compete with other industries for some classes of employees, have not been able to offset the same proportion of salary increases with productivity gains [112, p. 36]. As a result, the costs and prices of hospital care rise faster than the costs and prices of most other goods and services. For the other health services a relative lack of responsiveness on the part of the supplies of factors of production may be a contributory factor to the price increases. Given also the increasing per capita use of services, steadily rising expenditures for health and medical care are conducive to a permanent climate of financial crisis for which one group or another is blamed.

Nonprofit motive. For a large sector of the health and medical care industry the profit motive is not relevant as an explanation of behavior. Voluntary (nonprofit) organizations under religious, ethnic, or community auspices play a major part in rendering hospital care. Provision of large masses of social capital under such auspices derives from the historical circumstances under which the modern hospital developed, namely, its religious or ethnic sponsorship, its origin as a combination of a pesthouse and a hostel for the wanderer, its use as a clinical training ground for physicians and other health personnel, and the traditional belief that nobody should make a profit from illness. Although physicians on the staff are free to admit, treat, and discharge patients, a hospital's responsibility to the community for the amount and the quality of services rendered is vested in a board of trustees, on which practicing physicians do not usually sit. The result is separation between authority and responsibility in the voluntary hospital's management.

The voluntary character of the hospital has created other problems. Historically, the hospital's labor force has received low wages, and hospital organizations have striven for—and obtained—exemption from labor relations laws and from coverage under social insurance legislation. Furthermore, in the absence of the profit motive, the criteria for efficient operation are not obvious (see Chapter V, Section C).

Medical service and education as joint products. Medical service is frequently produced jointly with medical education and sometimes also with medical research. Most authorities believe that by conducting a good educational program a hospital enhances the quality of care rendered to its patients, since a teaching atmosphere and the presence of students foster curiosity and challenge practitioners to achieve their best performance [227, p. 8].

There is also a dissenting view, which notes that the interests of the physician and of the patient do not always coincide. For the former increased knowledge constitutes an important professional advance. For the latter scientific advances are not significant until they contribute to improved health [20, p. 120].

Costs tend to be higher in a teaching hospital than in a nonteaching hospital. From time to time it has been proposed that the costs attributable to education be segregated. In the past much of medical (including nursing) education was costless to the hospital; today an appreciable cost is entailed [132, pp. 239–40]. Only recently, with the assignment of house staff to private patients, has the value of their services to the practicing physician assumed significance.

Certain consequences of producing medical service and medical education jointly are perhaps less obvious. The educational element is certainly one reason why social capital has been provided in the hospital without charge to members of an independent profession who earn a good part of their living there. (Although assessments on medical staff members during hospital fund-raising drives are frowned upon, they are not uncommon.)

It is perhaps surprising that coupling of education and service may pose an obstacle to regional coordination of services. Almost all hospitals, not just the big medical centers, take pride in their teaching programs. Every physician concerned with teaching wants continuing access to good clinical material and is reluctant to part with patients who can be used for teaching, even when no fee is involved. It seems that his cooperation could be enlisted only if he were allowed to move with the patient, that is, if he had a staff appointment in more than one hospital.

The emphasis on good clinical material (which is often equated with acutely ill patients) may contribute to the relative neglect of services for patients with long-term illness or patients without exotic illness. Every teaching hospital is as selective as possible in admitting patients. Local government hospitals have less leeway to screen and choose than those under voluntary auspices and may become "dumping grounds." It has been suggested (by the writer's students) that the proximity of large government hospitals may be an essential prerequisite for the exercise of selectivity by other hospitals. In turn, the latter are enabled to give care of higher quality.

The tradition of using the poor for teaching purposes creates a problem when prosperity and health insurance combine to reduce the volume of the available clinical material. Sometimes an institution is reluctant to reduce ward and outpatient services, despite a decline in demand. Although the use of private patients for teaching is often discussed, it does not lend itself readily to the assumption of progressively increasing responsibility by house staff, especially by residents in surgery.

The list of distinctive economic characteristics of health and medical services can be summarized as follows: the irregular, uncertain, and sometimes communicable nature of illness; special attitudes of the public toward health and medical care; certain unusual characteristics of the inputs and outputs;

and unusual forms of organization in the provision of such services.

The personal experience of the economist also seems to constitute a problem in his dealings with the health field. Almost every economist who has expressed views on health and medical care has had some exposure to physicians and hospitals, personally or through his family or friends. His reaction is either strongly favorable or unfavorable; it is seldom neutral. Sometimes he comes to share Lady Mary Wortley Montagu's view of the physician as a person who would rather not eliminate smallpox lest his income drop. There is no greater knave in literature than Jules Romains' Dr. Knock.

Like most citizens the economist is impressed by technical advances in medicine and tends to accept at face value the claims of modern medicine to diagnose and treat illness and even to prevent it. As a result, he tends to view the absence of medical intervention as a deprivation, rather than as a possible form of "conservative" treatment designed to help nature along [30, p. 4]. Such subjective elements do not pervade the many other areas in which the economist works.

II. FACTORS INFLUENCING
DEMAND

In studying the economic aspects of health and medical services one is tempted to borrow the framework of the "medical care" field and to present the material under the headings of needs, personnel, facilities, organization, and finances. For an economic analysis it may, however, be more appropriate to employ the traditional framework of economics and to classify data and hypotheses under the factors comprising the demand for and supply of the product of an industry. This approach is most appropriate when the forces affecting demand and supply are distinct [11, p. 14].

Supply is defined and explained in Chapter IV. An analysis of the demand for an economic good begins with a statement about the probable relationship between price and quantity. The relationship is represented graphically by the demand curve, which typically slopes downward to the right—in other words, the quantity taken varies inversely with price. The demand curve rests on certain given factors: income, the prices of other goods, and tastes or preferences.

A. PRICE AND QUANTITY RELATIONSHIPS

It has been suggested that the demand for physicians' services is a demand for practitioners and not for specified units of service. The important economic relationship is not between the price and quantity of a given service but between the amount of money that individuals are willing to spend for medical care and the number of practitioners [124, pp. 157–58]. In determining the types and the amounts of care a patient requires, the physician may consider substituting inexpensive for costly services when inexpensive services are deemed capable of achieving the same result.

Application of a sliding scale of fees in the provision of physicians' services suggests that price has not performed here one of its ordinary market functions, namely, that of rationing a given supply among customers. A physician may provide the same service to different persons and charge them different prices, in accordance with his evaluation of the individual's ability to pay. He can do this because a medical service is not transferable between persons. Separation between consumer markets with different price elasticities of demand can, therefore, be maintained [43b, pp. 215–16]. (Price elasticity of demand is the percentage change in the quantity of a good taken by buyers associated with a 1 percent change in price. Because the relationship is inverse, price elasticity is negative.)

A sliding scale of fees is an old tradition in medicine. The medical profession views it as proof of its benevolent motives and professional (nonbusiness) standards of behavior. Many economists cite a sliding scale of fees as a classic instance of price discrimination [33, p. 180; 37, pp. 408, 425; 43b, pp. 219–20] and accept it only because it enables the poor as well as the rich to have access to the best physicians in a community. It is one of the informal, perhaps erratic, devices for equalizing income [81, p. 348]; unfortunately, the redistribution is limited to the sick [5, p. 26]. Other economists see a sliding scale of fees as evidence of monopolistic behavior [74, p. 20], as a means for maximizing the income of the medical profession [136, pp. 61–62]. Given, however, the low (less than one) price elasticity of demand for physicians' services (see p. 25 below), price discrimination cannot yield maximum profits [55, p. 957].

There is no denying that a sliding scale of fees has been effective in making most physicians in a community accessible to persons from different income classes. Indeed, owing to the limitations on outside practice imposed on full-time teachers in some medical schools, the well-to-do, rather than the poor, may be barred from receiving the best medical care.

If a sliding scale of fees were operative with respect to an individual's willingness to pay for care, as well as with respect to ability to pay, price would play no role whatsoever;

the quantity of services taken would be determined by medical needs as seen by the physician; and the demand function would be perfectly inelastic (the demand curve would be vertical). In practice the adjustment for ability to pay was probably less than perfect, being determined more often by a person's status than by his income, and the allowance for willingness to pay was probably erratic, depending on the physician's own attitudes.

The tradition of free care for the poor has nurtured medical education in the wards and outpatient departments of hospitals. Certain difficulties have arisen with the growth of voluntary health insurance. Regardless of what other effects it may produce, health insurance is designed to and does enhance an individual's ability to pay for the insured service. If the sliding scale is fully operative, the presence of insurance serves to raise the physician's fee, thereby vitiating the insurance benefit and wasting the purchaser's premium. Enough instances have been reported to suggest that some physicians are influenced by the presence of insurance to raise their fees [42, p. 202; 75b, p. 35]. Garbarino reports, however, that for one group of employees he studied, an increase in insurance benefits did not lead to a significant increase in physicians' charges [63, p. 76]. Whatever the facts may be, a sliding scale of fees is not compatible with health insurance financed by uniform premiums: if price discrimination with respect to benefits were perfect, the insurance would be worthless.

Authoritative opinion [42, p. 53; 63, p. 256], supported by some facts, holds that a sliding scale of fees is not so widely applied today as formerly. For example, a surgeon may charge a hospitalized patient one of two prices, depending on whether the patient occupies a private or a semiprivate bed.

Standardization of fees in a community is furthered by the movement toward relative value scales, which has been sponsored by a number of medical societies across the nation. Such scales assign specified weights to certain physicians' services, on the basis of a consensus among physicians. Given the price of an office visit (one unit), the prices of all other services are determined. In principle, individual physicians may differ in their basic unit price. To the extent that the office visit car-

ries a customary price (modal or typical, and slow to change),
all other fees tend to be more uniform then they would otherwise
be. (A tendency toward uniformity is also promoted through fee
schedules promulgated by large-scale purchasers of medical
service, such as government agencies or Blue Shield plans;
these may or may not apply the concept of the relative value
scale.)

In setting his standard fee, the physician is more likely to
be guided by tradition than by any estimate of the price elasticity of demand [120, p. 33]. Early in his career the physician
may have slack time, but he wishes to avoid being tagged by
his colleagues as a price cutter. After his career is well established, a rise in fees may fail to discourage clientele. Indeed,
the opposite may occur, if the new fee is sufficiently high to
carry prestige. (For a prestige good the demand curve slopes
upward to the right.)

In an emergency the patient and his family are inclined to
act as if price were no object. Patients tend to overcommit
themselves financially, and some doctors and hospitals regard
it as their social responsibility to protect patients and their
families against self-impoverishment. This attitude is one reason that some patients with hospital care insurance receive care
in the ward service [174, p. 135].

Hospitals usually charge three rates, based on the patient's
accommodation: private, semiprivate, and ward. The difference
between the first two categories reflects the degree of privacy—
and sometimes also a difference in the amenities of service—
and the difference between them and the ward service pertains
to the patient's ability and willingness to pay a physician. It
is intended that the semiprivate patient pay the hospital approximately the cost of care, that the charge to the private patient yield a net gain, and that the ward patient pay as much as
he can but no more than the cost to the hospital.

The growth of voluntary health insurance in this country
has been accompanied by an increase in the number and proportion of semiprivate hospital patients and by corresponding declines in ward and private patients. Simultaneously there has
occurred a marked rise in hospital patient day cost. As it be-

came less practical to finance a substantial proportion of ward care from net gains derived from charges to private patients, the percentage difference between private and semiprivate rates was allowed to decline. Ward patients have increasingly become the responsibility of government, which is expected to pay full cost. (Hospitals insist that government pay rates at full cost, regardless of the volume of services for which it pays [174, p. 372]. It would almost seem as if the goal were to maximize price rather than revenue. Such behavior is rational if hospitals prefer to retain freedom of action in setting rates for patients who are not certified as public charges.) Since government has insisted that its rates of payment must not exceed those quoted to self-paying patients, stated ward rates have risen faster than any other medical care price.

A lower rate may serve to attract patients to a hospital if their physician is associated with several hospitals and offers his patients a choice among them. This situation obtains most frequently in maternity care, when charges are stated in the form of an inclusive rate per stay. For medical and surgical care the consumer is faced with a multiplicity of rates for ancillary services as well as the charges for room and board. He is not likely to estimate correctly the probable total charges at each hospital, nor is he likely to think that he can do this. Indeed, even if average daily charges could be compared, differences in medical practice among hospital staffs might possibly result in offsetting differences in duration of stay. To the patient who is insured for service benefits, differences in hospital charges (or costs) are obviously of no concern. Moreover, many physicians are effectively associated with a single hospital, so that their patients lack the choice of a hospital. All of these considerations suggest that the demand for hospital care is not likely to respond to variations in price. (Robertson agrees with this broad conclusion but believes that demand may become more elastic after the acute phase of illness has passed and if the price rise is appreciable [89, pp. 45, 47]. Greenfield believes that demand is inelastic with respect to price changes, because most visits to physicians and hospitals are for curative services [14, p. 15]).

It is concluded that by and large, and within a reasonable range of prices, the quantity of physician services or hospital services demanded is not very responsive to price changes. (This conclusion is supported by Feldstein's recent calculations of price elasticity: 0.2 for physicians' services and 0 for hospital use [62, pp. 34, 40].) According to the above argument, the relative inelasticity is attributable less to the technical characteristics of the services (their essentiality at certain times) and more to the institutional (social, cultural, organizational) arrangements under which they are furnished. Perhaps many medical services are postponable or even dispensable [43b, p. 48]; even so, the market demand for them is inelastic under prevailing forms of medical care organization and pricing.

B. LEVEL OF DEMAND FUNCTION

The demand curve relates the quantities taken of a good to alternative prices, when other things are constant. Let us consider separately the effect on the level of demand for medical care when changes occur in (a) consumer income, (b) the price of medical care relative to the prices of other goods, and (c) consumer tastes or preferences. Included under the latter are a person's state of health and his perceptions of and attitudes toward medical care [62, p. 59].

Income

The amount of money a family spends for medical care increases with its income, but the proportion of its total income spent for medical care declines [53, pp. 17–18; 71, pp. 154, 159]. Some portion of the relatively high medical care expenditures at low incomes may reflect a temporary loss in family income due to the breadwinner's illness; some of it undoubtedly reflects a large volume of maternity and pediatric services used by young (low income) families [198, p. 23]; and some of it would reflect above average utilization by the aged (see p. 29 below). Apart from the young and the old, the poor have a higher incidence of illness than the rest of the population and require more care;

one obvious example is the incidence of tuberculosis and another is that of the diseases associated with high infant mortality.

The rise in absolute (dollar) expenditures for medical care as family income increases reflects in part the heavier use of certain services, such as dental care, and larger expenditures for some services that the well-to-do buy in greater quantities than the poor, such as private duty nursing. Probably, though not certainly, involved are both the operation of a sliding scale of fees, whose range has been narrowing, and the purchase of more expensive hospital accommodations and physicians' services by the well-to-do [14, p. 16; 55, p. 950]. In some geographic areas with inadequate local health resources, families with a high income are in a position to travel elsewhere for care, so that they also use more of the basic services, including those of physicians and hospitals, than the rest of the population.

Stigler has calculated the income elasticities of urban families for certain categories of health and medical services. (The income elasticity of demand is the percentage change in the quantity of medical services taken by buyers associated with a one percent change in income [43b, p. 50]. In the calculations expenditures are substituted for services. Only if prices are unchanged are the two concepts synonymous.) For physicians' services income elasticity is less than one and for dentists' services more than one. For other health and medical care elasticity declined from more than one in 1919 to less than one in 1941 [44, p. 27]. Stigler also calculated income elasticities for physicians' services by income class from data for the year 1935–36. The elasticity in each income class, as well as the average for all classes, was less than one, but it rose with income from 0.52 at $1,000 to 0.81 at $4,000 [43b, p. 52]. Using 1958 household survey data, Feldstein recently calculated an income elasticity of 0.6 [62, p. 75]; this may be too low [85, pp. 6, 386], because the measure of income is actual income rather than normal or permanent income.

Paradiso, using a time series of aggregate statistics (total consumer expenditures on an item, year by year) classified all consumer expenditure categories as "insensitive," "somewhat

sensitive," or "sensitive," depending on the size of the coefficient of income elasticity.   Before World War II private expenditures for physicians, hospitals, and private duty nurses
were "insensitive" to income changes and those for all other
medical care categories as classified by the U. S. Department
of Commerce were "somewhat sensitive" [7a, pp. 82, 723].
After the war expenditures for hospitals became "sensitive,"
but those for all other categories remained unchanged.   In the
late 1950s, however, expenditures for all categories of medical
care turned "sensitive."   The reason, Paradiso states, is that
the coefficients now reflected growth relationships almost exclusively rather than sensitivity to fluctuations in income [82,
pp. 28–29].

For more than twenty years private expenditures for medical
care in the United States remained a constant proportion of all
expenditures by consumers.   In the past decade, however, a rise
in the proportion has taken place.   Since the proportion of consumer expenditures to personal income has been constant for
many years, the proportion of medical care expenditures to aggregate personal income has been either constant or rising.   The
question is how to reconcile a constant or rising proportion of
medical care expenditures to income in the aggregate national
statistics with a declining proportion of medical care expenditures to family income in household survey data, as income increases.   The answer appears to be twofold.   One is technical,
having to do with fluctuations in family income from year to
year.   The other lies in the possibility of a shift in consumer
preferences or of changes in the relative prices of goods and
services.

Amidst fluctuations annual income is not so reliable a
measure of a family's standard of living or even of its long-run
average level of income as are its annual expenditures [99, p.
273].   Indeed, the few household surveys that present data on
medical care expenditures in relation to total family expenditures show a relatively constant proportion for all expenditure
classes, and even a slight increase in the upper classes [14,
p. 19; 71, pp. 151, 159].   Unfortunately, few surveys of consumer expenditures for health and medical care classify families

by expenditure class, and there are no recent ones. It is likely that the relationship would be even more positive if a family's normal income were substituted for total expenditures [85, p. 383].

Relative Prices

In continuation of a long-term trend [73, p. 130], the proportion of family income spent for medical care rose in every income class between 1953 and 1958 [53, p. 18]. The rise in price of a good with low price elasticity might be sufficient to account for this phenonenon. However, the possible contributions of a shift in consumer preferences toward health and medical care and of a change in relative prices between health and medical care and other goods and services should not be overlooked.

In the past decade the rise in medical care prices has outstripped the rise in prices of other major components of the Consumer Price Index [211, p. 1]. Other things being equal, an increase in the price of one good relative to the prices of other goods may be expected to lead to an attempt to substitute the other, now less costly, services. This tendency does not operate appreciably when the price elasticity of demand for the good in question is low, as it is for most components of medical care [62, p. 76]. The result of the greater rise in the prices of medical care is a greater rate of increase in expenditures for medical care than for other goods. The effect is magnified if the ratio of actual prices (payments) to stated prices for medical services rises as the collection ratio improves.

Perhaps more important in the demand for hospital care is one of the effects of health insurance, namely, the creation of a differential between the price of a good and the out-of-pocket expenditures by the consumer. It is possible for the prices of medical care to rise relative to the prices of other goods while the ratio of the out-of-pocket charges to other prices is declining. If so, the tendency would be to substitute medical care for other goods.

It has been suggested that a rise in the price of urban land

has led to the renting of smaller apartments. In turn, this has
led to the increased use of hospitals [51, p. 140].

Consumer Preferences

Considered here under preferences are two phenomena: a
true change of tastes or preferences on the part of a person; and
a shift in the composition of population toward groups with
above-average utilization of medical care.

Illustrative of the latter are the aged, who use larger amounts
of most types of medical service than younger persons [172, pp.
12–14, 78]. The proportion of aged persons in the population
has been rising. Particularly noteworthy is the differential behavior of the "older aged" (75 years old and over), who use
many more services than the "younger aged" (65–74 years) and
whose numbers are increasing at a higher rate [172, pp. 78, 80].

A question exists whether the association between high
hospital use and old age does not mask the effect of the loss of
a spouse [52, p. 70]. The fact remains that among the aged the
proportion of widowed is high, expecially among women. If the
widening differential between the sexes in life expectancy at
the older ages leads to a further increase in widowhood, it may
prove to be a more important factor than aging in increasing the
demand for institutional care.

The impact of aging on the use of long-term facilities may
be mitigated somewhat in the future, if the ability of able-bodied
aged persons to stay in the community improves. Owing to the
increase in social security benefits and private pensions, their
financial position has improved. Erection of public housing
may serve as partial replacement of domiciliary facilities in
institutions [172, p. 40].

The use of medical services tends to vary directly with the
level of education. The better educated are more health-conscious
and have a more positive attitude than the less educated toward
the early, and preventive, use of services [185, pp. 197, 209].
(It is conceivable that the early use of services may later lead
to a reduction in total services used; this argument is offered
by Feldstein to explain his finding that in the 1958 nationwide
household survey medical care expenditures are negatively

correlated with education [62, p. 64].) The same is true of urban populations, compared with rural populations [51, pp. 138–40].

Improvements in the environment and in medical care have effected a reduction in death rates in every age group, but this development is not necessarily accompanied by a lower use of medical care. Some current survivors have succeeded in avoiding illness altogether, with or without effort on their part. Some survivors became ill but regained their health and no longer require medical care. Others became ill and have not been by any means cured, but are able to function with support from physicians' services and drugs. (Good examples are diabetics and patients with rheumatic heart disease.) Other survivors have been recipients of prolonged life associated with prolonged illness or disabiltiy. (Examples are paraplegics and patients who require continuous maintenance rehabilitation.) These changes involve trading a reduction in mortality rates for a rise in morbidity (sickness and injury) [15, p. 91] and anxiety [30, p. 35]. At a given point of time a population may have a higher illness rate subsequent to medical progress than it would have had without such progress [32, p. 142; 77, p. 8].

As for the behavior of individuals, it appears that the public has gained increasing confidence in the efficacy of medical care to achieve cures. True, the public remains reluctant to undergo routine physical examinations, even when these are available without direct charge. However, the public's interest in the scientific aspects of medical care and its large stake in medical research have served to raise its expectations of medical care. The aspirations of people are more likely to be fulfilled today than formerly: if not for prevention, then for treatment; if not for cure, then for alleviation of pain and suffering.

All these factors lead one to expect an increase in per capita use of health and medical services. This is known to have occurred. In thirty years physicians' visits doubled (from 2.5 to 5 per person), and short-term hospital patient days rose almost 50 percent (from 860 to 1,265 per 1.000 population).

Voluntary health insurance has contributed to the increase (upward shift) in demand in several ways. One has been noted, namely, the creation of a differential between the price of a service and the out-of-pocket charge to the patient. Other ways in which health insurance serves to expand funds for payment are presented in the next section.

C. HEALTH INSURANCE

Health insurance is intended to facilitate the financing of medical care. Three fourths of this country's population have some form of voluntary health insurance. In the fiscal year 1961 premiums of $6.3 billion accounted for 22 percent of total health and medical care expenditures [76, Table 3]. Health insurance benefits are of major importance in paying for short-term hospital care (more than one half), of less importance in paying the doctor bill incurred in the hospital, and of still less importance in paying the doctor bill outside the hospital. Other health and medical services are not covered by insurance or are covered only to a small extent [53, p. 73].

The justification for health insurance is the uneven and unpredictable incidence of illness, which leads to wide fluctuations in individual and family expenditures for medical care over time and to extreme differences among individuals and families at a given time. Savings accumulated by a given date may prove to be insufficient to pay for an episode of illness. Health insurance can make the funds prepaid by a group of individuals and families sufficient to pay for the costs of covered illness during a specified interval. It is also the purpose of health insurance to equalize the distribution of the burden of medical care costs among individuals and families. If sold at a fair price and not vitiated by the operation of a sliding scale of fees, insurance is economically advantageous to the consumer, for it is a relatively painless way of saving for a rainy day and protects one's standard of living against adversity at a small calculable cost [36a, p. 580]. Health insurance also assures the producer of the receipt of payment for services rendered.

Increase in Utilization and in Expenditures
Even if one agrees that insurance is "a mechanism with a

limited objective and a limited function" [77, p. 674], it does not follow that insurance is without side effects [77, p. 673; 92, pp. 681–82]. Health insurance may be expected to increase the utilization of those services that are covered by it, as one barrier to the seeking of care is lowered or removed. Persons who are reluctant to ask for free care or lack access to it are now in a position to have it paid for. Initially an increase in the use of services is always in order, if only to correct prior neglect, and does in fact occur [52, pp. 42–45]. It is anticipated that ultimately the use of services will decline as the backlog of neglect is eliminated and as preventive medicine presumably bears fruit. However, the converse is also possible as subscribers become educated and learn to appreciate the benefits to which they are entitled and as receipt of insured services leads to the discovery of a need for and prescription of other services.

Surveys of hospital utilization agree on at least one finding: people with insurance enter the hospital more often and use more days of care on the average than do the uninsured [90, pp. 12–14]. One study shows that introduction of more complete benefits in a hospital insurance contract leads to an increased use of ancillary services [101, p. 130]. Other studies have shown greater "abuse" of hospital care by the insured than by the uninsured. (What constitutes "abuse" is a matter of controversy. The range of opinion is wide: hospital use as a function of the standard of living, at one end [153, p. 3], to hospital use as a medical phenomenon, capable of precise prescription, at the other end [Dr. Beverly Payne in 188, p. 5]. Classifications of abuse have been presented [96, pp. 171–82].) In part this finding reflects the selective impact of health insurance on the several types of health and medical service. Whenever an insured service (say inpatient care) and an uninsured service (say ambulatory care) compete as potential substitutes for one another, the insured service is likely to be preferred by the patient and condoned by the physician. (In addition to the technical substitutability of one service for another, it may be that the physician can expect to collect his own bill more easily and more certainly if other expenditures are met by insurance.)

If the insured service happens to be the more costly one, as in the case of hospital care, total expenditures for medical care are higher than they would otherwise be.

Health insurance entails a transfer of purchasing power from the well to the ill, thereby increasing the total demand for services [55, p. 943]. Expenditures for medical care are increased when some persons are removed from the ranks of the medically indigent and previously free services become paid for; or if the insurance benefit furnishes a new—and higher—base line for setting charges.

Insurance may lead to an increase in expenditures if incentives toward efficiency are impaired. It is conceivable that the restraint on cost increases is less when producers of hospital service are reimbursed at cost by insurance plans than when patients pay for care directly. Conversely, it may be that large purchasers of care are in a superior position to raise questions concerning proposed increases in premium.

Although it seems plausible that an insured population would spend more on medical care than an uninsured, there was no indication of the size of the differential before 1953, when Anderson and Feldman published their first report on family expenditures for medical care in the presence of insurance. As expected, they found that families with insurance incur higher total charges than families without insurance. Not so expected was the finding that the insured families also incur higher out-of pocket charges. The latter finding is reported at every income level [54, p. 26].

In 1953 families with insurance averaged out-of-pocket charges of $192. If an insurance premium of $56 is allowed for, the average (mean) cost to families with insurance was $248, whereas the average cost to those without insurance was $154.

If insured and uninsured families had the same characteristics in all other respects, one would expect the insured group to incur the smaller out-of-pocket charges. What accounts then for the unexpected direction of the difference?

One possible explanation is that the employer contribution toward health insurance premiums enables the employee to spend more for medical care. This may be partly true; but the average value of the employer contribution in 1952–53 could not have exceeded 20 percent of the premium, or $11 [75b, p. 29]. Hence the premium cost to the consumer was at least $45; this was in addition to the mean difference of $38 in out-of-pocket charges ($192 for the insured and $154 for the uninsured).

A second possibility is that the insured are charged higher fees, so that the value of their insurance benefit is partly vitiated. This explanation could apply to hospital care only in a very limited sense, namely, that the insured no longer receive free care and that some insured patients seek private, rather than semiprivate, accommodations. Some physicians, it is reported, raise the fee upon learning that the patient carries insurance. The fact that in 1953 the average family charge for surgery was higher for the uninsured than for the insured does not disprove this allegation; a lower average fee per procedure for the insured is consistent with their having a higher proportion of minor, less expensive, operations. Nevertheless, it is a striking fact that in every income class a higher proportion of persons with hospital care insurance than those without it received dental care [54, p. 200], which is not an insured service.

A third possibility is that insurance leads to the "abuse" of benefits. It is true that persons with insurance use more insured services than do uninsured persons; but it is also true that the former use more uninsured services, such as dental care. As for hospital care, the difference in utilization between insured and uninsured disappears in the $5,000-and-over income class; it may be that in the lower income classes the insured use the amount of care they need while the uninsured use less that an adequate amount. Even so, the pattern of hospital use in the higher income classes is different, with the insured having the higher rate of admission and the shorter average duration of stay. Also pointing toward the possibility of "abuse" is the fact that the small proportion of persons with two or more insurance policies have a higher hospital admission rate than those with a single policy. However, the adverse selection of risks may be a factor, too; that is, persons in poor health may be more inclined to secure multiple coverage than persons in good health.

A fourth possibility (suggested by Rashi Fein) is that under insurance the price of a service to the patient is so much lower than in the absence of insurance that a larger quantity of services may be used. If so, some out-of-pocket expenditures are usually entailed.

A fifth possibility is that the insured have both superior appreciation of and ability to pay for health and medical care. Consider the behavior of insured and uninsured individuals. The dollar difference between the expenditures of individuals is, of course, smaller than in the case of families; but it also does not follow the same pattern. Among individuals the insured and uninsured attain equal expenditures in the top income class; here the difference in medical expenditures between insured and uninsured families reflects size of family, not expenditure level. The difference between insured and uninsured individuals does, however, persist in all lower income classes. These facts are consistent with the view that above a certain income the appreciation of medical services is equally high among the insured and uninsured, and that the appreciation can be manifested through expenditures.

In light of the above it seems reasonable to suggest that persons with insurance are perhaps in a position to spend more money on most things, including uninsured medical services, in full knowledge of the protection afforded to them in the event of serious illness. With the risk of large expenditures reduced, they feel able to increase current consumption. In the course of time they become accustomed to a rising level of expenditures and seek to sustain it. The insured spend more than the uninsured because they want to, not because they have more illness and need more medical care. All known characteristics of the two groups point to this. With group enrollment so predominant in this country, there is little reason to believe that the enrollment process yields an adverse selection of risks.

It would be interesting to perform an empirical test of the validity of the last explanation. To begin with, are the reputed differences in charges real, or do they reflect differences between urban and rural cost levels? Since the difference in charges between the insured and uninsured holds true for each type of residential location [54, p. 118], geography appears not to be a factor. It should be possible to ascertain whether families with health insurance spend a higher proportion of their income than uninsured families and save less. (Alternatively, higher expenditures for medical care may be offset by lower expenditures for other goods and services.) It would also be interesting to observe the behavior of families in the course of time as they acquire insurance, hold it, and become accustomed to it.

Selected Problems

The retention charge of health insurance plans (premiums not paid out as benefits) obviously constitutes an addition to medical care expenditures. For many years the over-all retention charge approximated one fifth of all premiums, but currently it is 15 percent. It varies by insurance plan from a low of 7 percent for the nonprofit Blue Cross plans to 47 percent for individual insurance purchased from commercial plans [31, p. 12]. It is a moot question whether insurance with so high a retention rate is worth buying or serves a social purpose. Yet, it is this type of insurance that predominates among those groups in the population who are least likely to carry insurance, namely, the aged, farmers, and low income recipients [75a, p. 33; 80, p. 286].

Prominent among possible ways of achieving savings in health and medical care expenditures is the lower hospital use by subscribers to prepaid medical group practice plans that provide comprehensive benefits [165, p. 32]. A number of comparative studies have been conducted, the most recent of which cast some doubt on the proposition. (These are discussed in Chapter VI, Section A.) From the State of Washington it is reported that extending insurance benefits to home and office calls by physicians in solo practice who are paid on a fee-for-service basis leads to increased utilization of physicians' services; however, most of the rise in expenditures is offset by a reduction in hospital use [78, p. 14]. The conclusion is that insurance costs do not rise astronomically and are controllable. This reinforces the finding in Windsor, Ontario, that, contrary to expectations, insurance for comprehensive services by physicians in the community is practicable under the prevailing patterns of medical organization (solo practice) and payment for medical services (fee-for-service) [59, pp. 230–31].

The prevailing health insurance pattern affords good coverage for short-term illness treated in the hospital.. There is considerably less protection against prolonged illness or against expenses incurred outside the hospital. Dental care and psychiatric care are seldom covered outside major medical insurance [9, p. 645].

Controversy as well as confusion surrounds the question whether health insurance should be regarded as insurance in the classical sense or merely as prepayment, that is, budgeting in advance [69, p. 49]. The practical issue is whether the cost of obstetrical care or a periodic health examination, each being foreseeable for the individual and family, is best paid for by the patient directly, without loading on the additional expense of processing the claim, or through an insurance plan, in recognition of the prevailing custom of purchasing most things on installment. The possibility of organized post-payment for medical care has not been seriously explored.

Since requirements for health services are not strictly defined by the patient's diagnostic condition, wide variation in the use of services is possible and even "abuse." Participation in payment by the patient—through a deductible amount or a coinsurance percentage—is intended to serve as a compromise between the incentive effects of insurance (the moral hazard factor) that may lead to misuse and the reallocation of risk-bearing through insurance that enhances consumer welfare [55, p. 961]. It has been observed that coinsurance is not a deterrent to extravagant spending by the well-to-do while it imposes excessive burdens on the average family [103, pp. 35–36].

Perhaps a coinsurance feature might be applied only to nonserious illness. An example would be cancellation of the supplementary payment by the patient if the cost of medical care exceeded a specified percentage of his income [77, p. 672]. A variant of this approach would be to confine supplementary payment to the room and board portion of a hospital stay, on the ground that this amount would be reasonably predictable; the use of ancillary services by patients displays far greater variation [193, pp. 170–71]. Rothenberg proposed a point rationing scheme that would distinguish between serious and nonserious illness [92, p. 686].

An objection to coinsurance is that it is incompatible with service benefits, under which the enrollee is assured of receiving without charge the services specified in the contract. In effect, the subscriber is insured against the uncertainty of price change, as well as against the uncertainty of need for services [55, p. 962]. The arguments for service benefits are two: with cash benefits some physicians cannot be trusted to charge their regular fees [69, p. 52]; and service benefits preclude the assumption of unlimited liability by the patient [91, p. 139]. Since the provision of specified services necessitates a contract between insurance plans and providers of service, the former are likely to move toward quantity and quality controls.

Since workmen's compensation benefits for medical care are not commonly considered in this context, health insurance in this country is almost always modified by the word "voluntary." A few have questioned the appropriateness of the adjective, observing that group enrollment and employer contributions exert strong pressures and incentives, respectively, for individuals to join.   Other students point to the possibly coercive effects exerted on more provident citizens by the refusal of some persons to buy voluntary insurance [92, p. 683; 125, p. 299]. In effect, their refusal is a gamble that in the event of illness they would receive a free ride as medically indigent patients.

The voluntary nature of health insurance has important consequences.   Premiums cannot be varied with income [80, p. 266]. Equal premiums, more or less, imply that among certain disadvantaged groups the proportion with insurance is low [80, p. 288], so that government and philanthropy must continue to participate in financing personal health services.   Another result is the persistence of a large number of diverse insurance plans (currently 1,800) none of which may occupy a predominant or even important position in a given geographic area.   A third result is the pressure on insurance plans that offer service benefits to keep premiums down [131, pp. 79–80]. Some of these plans respond with one or another form of experience rating, in contrast to the application of a uniform community-wide premium [80, p. 193].

There is some question regarding the extent to which one can rely on voluntary health insurance to finance health and medical care for the aged (65 years and over). The task is complicated by these facts: (a) the incomes of aged persons decline or cease; (b) their use of health and medical services exceeds that of the rest of the population; and (c) voluntary health insurance, especially at group premiums, is not so readily available to them.

The proportion of aged persons who hold some form of health insurance rose from 26 percent in 1952 to 55 percent in 1963. However, they encounter obstacles in purchasing insurance with substantial benefits. Conversion from group to individual insurance involves a rise in premium and sometimes also a reduction in benefits. For members of nonprofit plans the rise in premium is of the order of 20 percent, because these plans apply the "community rate," through which the cost of providing extra services to the aged is spread among the younger 90 percent of the population. For subscribers to commercial insurance the increase in premiums may be as high as 200 to 300 percent [75b, p. 39]. For some retirees the additional cost is superimposed upon the withdrawal of the employer contribution to the premium.

Currently advocated is a proposal to employ the Old Age, Survivors, and Disability Insurance (Social Security) Trust Fund for insuring the aged for certain health and medical services on a complusory basis. Hospitalization and nursing-home benefits would be the points of departure, just as under voluntary insurance, with physicians' services actually excluded. This is an undesirable bias [86, p. 114].

Hitherto Old Age and Survivors Insurance has been confined to cash benefits for income maintenance. If extended to the health field, the objective of the insurance would be to provide and pay for specified services. This is a significant difference.

It means that the insurance fund must develop close relationships with the producers of services. To the extent that the
cost of hospital care continues to rise at a faster rate than other
costs and payrolls (see Chapter V, Section B), a given sum
actuarially calculated today and set aside over the next generation or two would prove insufficient to buy a specified set of
services.

Weighing heavily in favor of affirmative action is the high
cost of health and medical care for the aged and their inability
to pay for it out of current income or assets. Prepayment during
one's productive life is necessary, as well as portability of ac-
crued benefits from one job to another. These requirements im-
pose serious constraints on our ability to solve the problem
without help from government. The latter hesitates to propose
legislation involving physicians' services lest the entire program
be jeopardized by the opposition of organized medicine.

III. DEMAND BY BUSINESS, PHILANTHROPY, AND GOVERNMENT

The theory of demand discussed in the preceding chapter applies to consumers. The demand curve of buyers in the market place is a function of prices, income, and preferences (which, in turn, represent a congeries of psychological wants and cultural aspirations). In paying for health services, however, the consumer's position is not the dominant one. In the fiscal year 1961 his expenditures constituted three fifths of all expenditures for health and medical care. His out-of-pocket payments accounted for less than one half of total expenditures [76, Table 3].

Sources of demand for health and medical services other than consumers are business and government, as in most fields of economic activity, and also philanthropy. This chapter deals with the several sources of demand. After outlining the implications of diversity, it will discuss health and medical care expenditures by business (section A); the case for intervention, that is, the reasons that philanthropy and government participate in financing health and medical care (section B); the role of philanthropic income (section C); and the uses of tax funds and various devices, such as deductions and exemptions (sections D and E).

Diversity in sources of payment for health and medical care has two facets. It may in itself lend an element of strength to the financial underpinnings of the industry [70]. Opposition to increases in expenditures is diluted. Economic power is dispersed, and experimentation in program may be encouraged. There is greater flexibility in meeting changing conditions, for at a given time one source or another may be in a superior position to raise funds. At the same time the burden of a given expenditure does not necessarily fall on a particular pocketbook. Under certain circumstances, especially when a cause is popular, the several sources of funds may actually compete to pay for services.

The other facet of diversity is complexity. It is by no means obvious when the consumer, business, philanthropy, or government will pay for a given set of services. (The major exception to an indeterminate answer is that in the event of an industrial injury workmen's compensation insurance supersedes other payment mechanisms.) It is a question of ability to pay plus opportunity to transfer the burden to another source of payment.

The source of payment is often associated, though not uniquely, with a particular payment mechanism. As a result, source of payment may affect the volume of services used and price, and, therefore, the amount of money spent.

A. EXPENDITURES BY BUSINESS

Business expenditures for health and medical care consist largely of three items: in-plant health services, medical benefits under workmen's compensation insurance, and contributions to voluntary health insurance in behalf of employees and their dependents. The last item has had the most rapid rate of growth in the postwar era and is now the largest component of business expenditures ($2.8 billion of a total of $3.5 billion estimated for fiscal year 1961) [76, Table 3].

Employer Contributions and Union Participation

From the very inception of the voluntary health insurance movement in this country in 1929 the enrollment of employee groups has been emphasized. During World War II wages were frozen, but increases in fringe benefits were permitted. These became subject to collective bargaining, and unions came to ask for and receive employer contributions in increasing amounts, first toward the premiums of employees and subsequently toward the premiums of dependents. Deductibility of employer contributions under the corporation income tax is a powerful social invention [63, p. 4].

Employer contributions are known to have increased in amount immediately after World War II, but the scattered evidence does not warrant the estimation of a figure. For the year 1951 the figure of 37.5 percent has been offered as the proportion of health insurance premiums contributed by employers [5, p. 307]. The figure of $750 million cited by Robertson for 1952 yields an even higher proportion, 45 percent or more [88, p. 57]. The first official estimate of employer contributions was prepared by Louis Reed for 1954. The writer published estimates for 1953 and 1955, which came to one quarter of all premiums [75b, p. 29]. Following the same methods the proportion for 1961 has been estimated at 44 percent [76, p. 64].

The $2.8 billion in question does not represent an addition of this amount to the sums that would otherwise be available to finance voluntary health insurance. In many instances an increase in the employer contribution has served to relieve the employee of his own payment. The employer contribution has also permitted an expansion of benefits with a constant employee payment, which might otherwise not have occurred (if only through avoidance of the tax on personal incomes). In some industries it has served to extend insurance to low-wage employees, some of whom would not have bought it with their own money. Moreover, any earmarking of funds establishes a floor for financing the designated program. It seems reasonable to suppose that the employer contribution has increased the sums available to finance health and medical care.

Health insurance for employee groups under private auspices does not entail the accumulation of substantial funds. Premiums equal benefits plus cost of administration (including reserves for pending maternity cases and for epidemics). In the absence of an accumulated fund, there is no occasion to grant portability rights. It suffices to assure the right to convert (without medical examination but perhaps at higher premium) from group to individual insurance. However, if retired persons are to be brought under voluntary health insurance, the accumulation of a fund and the granting of portability rights to employees appear to be necessary.

Employment status is an important factor in determining an individual's or family's insurance status and may overtake income as the overriding influence. However, the employer contribution is not available to the unemployed, most retired persons, and domestic servants—groups that are in greater need of a supplementation of income than those to whom it is now available. At the same time, by paying somewhat higher prices for the goods the others produce (owing to partial shifting of the contribution to consumers) [39, p. 306], the unemployed and the aged participate in financing health insurance for the employed and the unionized. The question has been raised whether the health insurance benefits now extended to some through employer contributions should not be made available to all through public intervention [65, p. 144].

Collective bargaining has brought the labor unions prominently into the health insurance field. They exert influence directly through participation in, or control over, the management of health and welfare funds and indirectly as a major representative of the consumer interest, serving as spokesman before the public and before state commissioners of insurance and as members of boards of directors of Blue Cross plans. A union exerts a greater measure of influence and control in industries with small firms where multiemployer health and welfare funds predominate.

A health and welfare fund can choose one of three courses of action: (a) to establish its own program of service; (b) to purchase care through an insurance plan; and (c) to purchase care through self-insurance. Though the third course has been urged upon unions as a conserver of funds, the second course is followed most commonly. The first course is often employed as a threat but seldom adopted, for the mere utterance of the threat frequently leads to an intensive courting of the union leaders by the existing producers of services.

A union that produces services is least likely to operate a hospital—miners living in isolated and poor communities were a notable exception—and most likely to establish a union health center. For the past decade and longer new union health centers in New York State have limited their activities to the provision of diagnostic services only. The reasons are as follows: a single facility is too centralized to provide treatment conveniently to all union members as they live in different parts of a large city or metropolitan area; the delivery of treatment services to ambulatory patients through organized facilities is opposed by medical societies and is, therefore, unlikely to pass the state legislature; and diagnostic services, especially periodic health examinations, can provide benefits for a large proportion of union members [63, p. 250].

In-plant Health and Medical Services

A decision to establish a program of in-plant health services is based on the ordinary profit and loss calculations of a firm, except in the case of firms in isolated communities. For a given expenditure a well-planned employee health program will presumably result in a reduction in illness on the job and absenteeism from the job. In turn, these will yield an increased output with the same or smaller size of the work force. It is recognized that the results of the calculation are influenced by factors other than employees' convenient access to health and medical services without charge, such as the firm's policy on sick pay. An in-plant health and medical program is frequently associated with a reduction in premiums for workmen's compensation insurance.

The cost of the program per employee declines as the number of employees in a plant increases. Accordingly, large plants are much more likely than small ones to operate in-plant health and medical programs. The cost of all such programs in the fiscal year 1961 is officially estimated at $0.3 billion [21, p. 10].

Workmen's Compensation

Workmen's compensation insurance is intended to protect employees against the hazards of occupational injury or sickness by providing them with medical care, as well as with cash benefits in lieu of earnings, without resort to litigation. The program constitutes a distinct source of payment for medical care with priority over other sources of payment, so that cases covered by workmen's compensation insurance are specifically excluded from benefits under voluntary health insurance. Because the expenditures are required by statute, the official figures classify them in the public sector. It is estimated that seven eights of all medical care expenditures under workmen's compensation are incurred by business and one eighth by government. In turn, the medical benefits of $0.4 billion in the fiscal year 1961 constitute almost one third of all benefits under workmen's compensation [21, p. 10].

Perhaps three fifths of the medical care benefits under workmen's compensation are spent for physicians' services [75a, p. 52]; information on this item is scanty. The quality of the care furnished by workmen's compensation physicians has long been a point of contention. Formerly the care was provided by contract physicians, but recently most states have allowed injured workers to choose their own physician. There is an element of irony in the situation; labor unions favor the free choice of a physician in workmen's compensation cases but frequently question its desirability under voluntary health insurance [84, p. 177]. Conversely, an official of the American Medical Association, which espouses the free choice of a physician under most circumstances, opposes it in workmen's compensation cases [95, p. 172].

Either method of providing physicians' services may lead to abuse: the contract physician system tends to skimp on services in order to reduce the cost of care, whereas the free choice system tends to steer the medical diagnosis, treatment, and prognosis toward a larger cash award. The problem is that the physician who is relied upon for medical care and rehabilitation services must also assist in determining the extent of the damage that has been sustained permanently. The absence of administrative supervision by a neutral party over the quality of medical care is widely regarded as a serious deficiency in a workmen's compensation program [84, p. 175; 194, pp. 59-60].

Hospitals receive two fifths of all medical care benefits under workmen's compensation. These payments constitute a small proportion (perhaps 2 percent) of the income of short-term hospitals. In New York state hospitals are paid promulgated room rates, which vary with the size of hospital, and also specified fees for ancillary services, which are the same as the fees paid to physicians in private practice for the same services.

The principal argument for a rehabilitation program under

workmen's compensation, aside from humanitarian considerations, is its economic benefits [95, p. 251]. Frequently listed benefits are the savings in relief payments to persons who have been rehabilitated; the increase in their output; and the rise in income tax receipts [93, p. 139].

Conley sees the taxes not paid during disability and the additional maintenance costs of the disabled financed through taxes as costs of disability to the rest of society [195, Chapter 2, p. 18]. The writer believes, however, that inclusion of relief payments and tax receipts constitutes double or even triple counting of the economic loss avoided through rehabilitation (see Chapter VII, Section B). Giving them separate recognition may, however, be pertinent to particular agencies or levels of government or business firms in deciding on their own expenditures.

Legislators, one is told, are not impressed by arguments regarding the economic benefits of rehabilitation, except during periods of intense manpower shortage, such as wartime [95, p. 254]. Such skepticism may be warranted, for in the past the market economy has apparently not absorbed appreciable numbers of rehabilitated persons [12, p. 736]. The best adjustment is made by workers who return to jobs in their old firms [194, p. 300].

B. THE CASE FOR INTERVENTION

The market mechanism is neither all pervasive in the health and medical care industry nor given full sway in the areas it does permeate. The question is: Why do government and philanthropy play such important parts in the provision and financing of health and medical services? In this section an attempt is made to bring together from the economic literature a systematic discussion of public intervention in the financing of such services.

No distinction is made here between intervention by government and intervention by philanthropy. A distinction, however, is made between collective sources of funds on the one hand and collective activities on the other hand [16, p. 113; 19, p. 19;

56, pp. 16, 113]. Although the practicability of divorcing
payment by government from production by government has been
questioned [60, p. 290; 185, p. 142], it seems indisputable to
the writer that there can be government expenditures without
government production (as in purchasing care for public assistance recipients in proprietary nursing homes) as well as
government production with some private payments (as in caring
for paying patients in hospitals associated with state medical
schools).

Perhaps it goes without saying that economic grounds for
intervention have meaning only within the context of customary
beliefs regarding the individual's or family's responsibilities
and of popular attitudes toward the exercise of authority by
government [3, p. 28]. Moreover, the relevant issue of state
action, like most issues in economic policy in this country, is
not one of "yes or no" but of "more or less" [27, p. 110].
Since one may regard governmental action as coercive in a way
that market action is not, governmental action may require the
erection of stronger safeguards [35, p. 72].

Almost two hundred years ago Adam Smith included the construction and maintenance of large public works among the three
duties of a sovereign [40, p. 651], the others being national defense and administration of justice. In this generation it has
been observed that the latter two activities differ from health
and medical care only in degree and that there were times in the
past when neither was the object of public concern and of collective action [37, p. 186].

Public Health and Medical Research

The case for the provision of "public health" services and
for the financing of medical research by government rests essentially on three grounds: (a) the special characteristics of
so-called collective (or public) goods; (b) external relationships
in consumption; and (c) declining unit cost of production [24,
p. 790; 27, p. 116; 56, pp. 91–100; 111, pp. 22–24; 208, p. 3;
229, pp. 16–27]. It is not always clear whether Weisbrod, who
employed this scheme, was referring to all health services, including personal medical care, or only to the traditional public

health services aimed at improving control over the environment, including efforts to limit the spread of communicable diseases.

Collective goods. A good is said to be collective (or public or social) if one person's consumption of it causes no diminution of what is left for others [94, p. 387]. "More for you means no less for me." The most frequently cited example of such a good is the lighthouse [56, p. 91]. Weisbrod's example from public health is the benefits that a group derives from a spraying campaign against flies and mosquitos [229, p. 17]. Often such a good cannot be appropriated by an individual [2, p. 19]; but though the characteristic of inappropriability is often present, it is not essential [56, p. 99]. The essential characteristic is that there be no way to exclude individuals from enjoying the good [23, p. 9].

Since the benefits of a spraying campaign against flies and mosquitoes would accrue equally to all residents of an area (an individual's consumption being a function of total supply, not of the quantity he buys), there is no incentive for anybody to volunteer and offer to pay for the service [23, p. 10]. Rather, there is a temptation to hide one's real preferences and to pretend lack of interest, in the hope that others who wish to enjoy the benefits of the program will offer to pay. There is, therefore, an apparent absence of demand, and financing through voluntary means is likely to be inadequate. More important, if collective goods are to be available for individuals to enjoy, it becomes advantageous to enlist the help of the coercive power of the state [58, p. 91].

A fluoridated water supply seems to be another example of a collective good. As long as there is an adequate quantity of water and if the engineers succeed in maintaining a uniform fluoride content, consumption by one does not deprive another. (This example was suggested by the writer's students.)

Medical research, especially the basic research component, is a similar product in the sense that new ideas can be used over and over without being consumed. Since the benefits of basic research are diffuse and the cost of reproducing research is much less than the cost of initially producing it [55, p. 946], there is little incentive for private enterprise to undertake it.

Under strictly private auspices basic medical research would be underfinanced [51, p. 141; 55, p. 946], and the need of government subsidy is evident [87, p. 138]. Where the benefits of medical research can be appropriated and private financing is forthcoming, serious issues arise concerning patent policy, control of monopolistic practices, and the utility of the research that is performed.

External effects in consumption. Certain health and medical services exert an appreciable effect on persons other than the immediate recipients. Consider a vaccination, which is a personal health service, in that it is administered to an individual. In case of a communicable disease the benefit of the vaccine extends not only to the person who receives it but also to members of the community who do not. (This effect should be distinguished from another important kind of external economy of consumption, namely, the satisfaction an individual may derive from improvement in the health of other persons, as well as in his own [56, p. 91]. Still another external relationship in consumption is "keeping up with the Joneses.") Thinking only of the benefits that accrue to himself, the price an individual would be willing to pay for his vaccination is lower than that which the community would be willing to pay [25, p. 4]. Accordingly, the values of the private and the social benefits diverge, and it would be advantageous for society to pay a subsidy to encourage vaccination.

External benefits also accrue from medical research. If an additional investigator learns of new findings, the probability of further advances is enhanced.

Declining unit cost. Some services can be obtained only by erecting large and costly facilities. Water works and sewage disposal plants are examples of facilities that cannot be economically built on a small scale; that is, the economist would say, the physical capital is not finely divisible [33, p. 334]. If the service is to be provided at all, a sizable capital investment is required.

In enterprises with large amounts of specialized resources fixed cost represents a high proportion of total cost at most outputs. Since such enterprises can be operated at declining unit cost, an increase in output is associated with reduced cost. The higher the ratio of fixed to variable cost, the larger is the range over which average cost falls [43b, p. 170; 56, pp. 93–94]. A service that would be expensive to produce for an individual or a small group could be cheap for a large group [229, p. 20].

Physical plants that require large capital investments produce services over many decades. An individual may see the distant future but dimly and is likely to prefer paying for services that will accrue shortly or during his own lifetime. When individual judgment is sovereign, that is, in the absence of public intervention, underinvestment is likely to take place [58, pp. 91–92; 111, p. 24].

Support of voluntary forms of organization. A fourth ground for interfering with the market mechanism in the health field is society's preference for facilities owned and operated under certain auspices, say voluntary (nonprofit) organizations, over facilities owned and operated under other auspices, say for profit [55, p. 950]. This preference for one form of organization over another is apart from, and in addition to, the pursuit of similar objectives through regulation by government or by voluntary agencies, such as professional societies (see Chapter V, Section C, and Chapter VI, Section D). The federal Hill-Burton program, which provides matching grants to help construct nonprofit hospitals, governmental or voluntary, reflects an effort to stimulate the growth of the nonbusiness sector of the hospital industry.

The case for intervention has received wide support in principle. There is considerable divergence of opinion concerning its implementation.

Even Lees, a severe critic of government action, agrees that clearing a malarial swamp or a polluted water supply constitutes provision of a public good [19, p. 18]. However, in his opinion most health and medical services are not public goods, in the sense of being consumed equally by all; rather, health services can be enjoyed by consumers separately, and increased consumption by some implies reduced consumption by others. Moreover, Lees sets narrow limits to the range of external benefits; he would include a public menace, such as an epidemic, but would exclude private misfortunes [213, pp. 33–34]. In the event of a public menace Lees would employ public subsidies to help pay for the provision of the requisite services by the private sector of the economy. The objectives of such subsidies are two-fold: (a) to reduce the cost of the service to the consumer and (b) to offer him incentives to resist any tendency to act perversely (against his true interest) or to minimize the risk of illness [19, p. 26].

It has been suggested that outside the realm of national defense, basic research, and the proverbial lighthouse, the category of collective good is likely to be small [57, p. 165]. Also pointing against intervention is the difficulty of measuring the value of external benefits. One book concludes: "In general, recognition in principle of a case for state intervention is not tantamount to a recommendation of policy measures, the implementation of which... may easily deviate far from the theoretical ideal and then be wasteful" [57, p. 166].

It has also been pointed out that the use of hospitals, even those owned and operated by government, must be rationed on some basis. It is simply not true at a given time that the use of a facility by individual A does not involve some cost to B. The justification of public expenditures on the ground that the benefit of a particular service cannot be appropriated by individuals is, in one opinion, of no help to the understanding of most public expenditures [81, pp. 347–48].

Personal Health Services

Numerous arguments have been adduced in favor of public intervention in financing personal health and medical services that are without important external effects. A common element is the desire to alter the results achieved by the market.

Importance of availability of health services. Without public intervention an important service may not be available in sufficient quantity in some geographic areas, owing to their inability to attract the necessary supplies of indivisible health personnel and facilities [55, p. 955]. Thus, one economist has suggested that in each area sufficient and accessible resources must be allocated to health and medical services to permit at least caring for all serious conditions. He defines such conditions as characterized by an almost perfectly inelastic demand for medical care, or by important neighborhood (external) effects, or by both [92, p. 677]. Another economist characterizes medical services as quasi-collective and recognizes the interest of government and philanthropy in the provision of hospital facilities and services [2, pp. 22, 400].

Assistance to the poor. For centuries hospitals were devoted exclusively to the sick poor. When hospital service was extended to the middle- and upper-income classes, continuing the provision of free services to the poor became one way to reduce inequality in the distribution of income. In theory, there is no reason why any advantages enjoyed by the wealthier classes in purchasing medical care cannot be overcome by redistributing income. In practice, however, not all redistribution does—or can—take place through taxes and transfer payments (government cash subsidies) [28, pp. 42–43; 81, p. 348].

At a given time persons with low income may have a greater need than other persons for services and a lesser ability to purchase them. Provision of certain personal health and medical services, especially rehabilitation services, could effect a return of the sick poor to economic self-sufficiency. Society would then benefit from the increase in output. Conversely, an appreciable proportion of expenditures for health and medical services is incurred in behalf of the aged, most of whom will not make a further contribution to production.

It has been suggested that, apart from the problem of the sick poor, the very uneven incidence of illness may be a cause of social concern [204, p. 284]. The effort to finance prolonged serious illness out of pocket can turn a well-to-do family into a medically indigent one, no longer able to pay all its medical bills at the accustomed level of charges.

Protection of government wards. In this country government assumes responsibility for the health and medical care of certain groups in addition to the poor. Among them are veterans, particularly those veterans who acquired disabilities in the service. Patients with mental illness have long been acknowledged as a public responsibility. Even Lees favors a role for government in caring for patients with mental illness and long-term illness, and in the provision of expensive drugs, though he offers no reasons [19, p. 56]. Care of patients with tuberculosis is also a responsibility of government, owing to the long duration of patient stay in the hospital (formerly much longer than today) and the contagious character of the disease.

Frequently health and medical services are provided to mothers and infants, giving them an extra measure of protection in their defenseless state. Children may be protected against the tendency by some parents to neglect the long-term interests of their offspring. Pigou holds that neglect of the interests of future generations may be one of the most serious disharmonies in a market economy [27, p. 116].

Unreliability of consumer's choice. In the health field social judgment is perhaps more generous than private judgment. In addition to a difference in purchasing power, society is not so inhibited by considerations of futurity (preference for current over future consumption), irregularity of payments for health and medical services on a fee for service basis, and the unpleasantness frequently associated with the receipt of medical care [65, p. 143].

These factors, plus the tendency of individuals to underestimate the risk of illness in the absence of symptoms, indicate that perhaps consumers spend too little for their own health and medical care. In a technically complex field, such as health services, perceived advantage and actual private advantage may diverge owing to the buyer's ignorance [111, p. 22]. If so, Clark would substitute the judgment of trained experts for that of consumers [161, pp. 128–29].

It has been suggested that the nation cannot afford to permit private decisions to determine expenditures on health and medical care any more than on education. Consumers need guidance, as shown by a comparison of the amounts they spend on medical care and on other things, such as tobacco, alcohol, personal care, and recreation [67, p. 310]. This is akin, on the one hand, to Dickinson's argument that consumers get as much medical care as they are willing to pay for [196, pp. 7–8, 12] and, on the other hand, to J. K. Galbraith's argument in *The Affluent Society* concerning an imbalance between private expenditures for outsized automobiles and the neglect of such useful things as hospitals. Consonant with the latter view is Hansen's belief that the marginal tax dollar has greater social utility than the marginal pay envelope dollar; in his opinion additional resources should be diverted to hospitals [16, p. 345].

A comparison of amounts spent on various items, however, can be misleading. Some may view expenditures for tobacco, liquor, or recreation as morally reprehensible, but for the individual consumer they are certain and regular in occurrence, low-priced per unit of purchase, and usually pleasurable. The amount spent for health and medical care is the sum of many small and some large expenditures. It remains to be shown empirically that persons with small expenditures for medical care indulge in large expenditures for liquor, tobacco, etc. [130, p. 639]. Lees states that the imbalance argument smacks of mysticism [213, p. 35]. Also to be taken into account is the value, if any, attached to free choice by the consumer in spending his income.

Effect on employment. It has been suggested that increased expenditures for health and medical care would provide employment for resources released from manufacturing [67, p. 321] and opportunities for a livelihood in the professions for the increasing numbers of college graduates [67, p. 315]. In the writer's opinion, to argue for increased public expenditures on these grounds is tantamount to assuming that a high rate of unemployment would otherwise persist or would be difficult to overcome. It is also implicitly assumed that the best—perhaps only—route to good health is through medical services (see Chapter IV, Section E).

In summary, the economic bases for public intervention in financing public health services are as follows: the nature of collective goods; the presence of external benefits; the decline of unit cost with increases in output; and society's preference for nonprofit forms of organization in the health field. With respect to personal health services, the reasons for intervention are the following: to assure the presence of some health personnel and facilities in a locality; to assist the sick poor, including the medically indigent; to protect certain groups who are government wards by tradition; to offset the working of consumers' choice, which is not reliable; and to increase employment outlets in the economy. Pervading both sets of arguments is a possible divergence in time preference between individuals and society, reflecting a difference between their attitudes toward the next and succeeding generations.

C. PHILANTHROPY

It has been noted that in the health field efforts to moderate or alter the results (or failures) of the market may take the form of collective action under voluntary (nonprofit) auspices [55, p. 948], as well as through government. On the demand side, philanthropic funds exert a small effect over-all but have substantial impact in certain areas, such as hospitals, visiting nurse services, and the national voluntary agencies for the control of specific diseases.

The factors responsible for the establishment of voluntary nonprofit hospitals in this country and, consequently, for donations to them are discussed in Chapter V, Section C.

Visiting nurse agencies offer nursing services in the home. Some also provide ancillary services, such as housekeeping, and a few supervise organized home care programs. Traditionally, visiting nurse services have cared for middle-income patients as well as the poor, charging fees according to patients' ability to pay and financing losses through income from philanthropic sources.

The national voluntary health agencies have become "big business" in the past two decades [66, p. 9]. Distinguished one from another by category of disease, they raise money from the public for the purpose of encouraging research, training, and health education in their respective fields.

Total Funds and Their Uses

Reported estimates of philanthropic funds always include cash contributions toward expenditures for current purposes.

Contributions for building are usually excluded or shown separately. Donations for other capital purposes may be counted in full, in part (excluding, for example, contributions toward endowment funds), or not at all. In the last situation earnings on investments may be reported in full or in part. Donated services are usually excluded, with the possible exception of the value of the contribution of full-time workers, most commonly members of religious orders.

Excluded from all measures of philanthropic contributions are the services of part-time volunteers serving as board members or rendering services to the sick. The services of lay volunteers are not counted, because the use of leisure time does not enter into the calculation of national income. For physicians the contribution of time to hospitals and clinics enhances their earning power. More important, the rendering of free care by physicians is so meshed with the way they charge fees and earn incomes, that it seems best to regard total expenditures for physicians' services as the market's evaluation of all services rendered, not only those paid for [75b, pp. 25–26]. Indeed, there is reason to believe that a sliding scale of fees leads to an increase in consumer expenditures for physicians' services by enabling physicians who draw patients from a wide range of economic classes to charge maximum fees to each [136, p. 61].

It is estimated that physicians allot one eighth of their time to free care [76, p. 40]. One source distributes the total amount of free care as follows: 40 percent to private inpatients, 23 percent in the outpatient department, 26 percent in hospital wards, and 11 percent to courtesy cases [97, p. 99]. Thus, approximately one half of all free care by physicians is extended to the poor.

The official (Merriam) estimates on philanthropic contributions for health and medical care exclude contributions toward hospital construction but are intended to include all other contributions of cash and property. The value of services donated by members of religious orders is excluded [66, pp. 60, 78]. To the published figure of $0.7 billion for the fiscal year 1961 [21, p. 10] may be added another $0.3 billion ($235 million for

construction and $60 million as donated services of Sisters)
[76, Table 10], yielding a total of $1.0 billion.

One study of national voluntary health and welfare agencies
found a paucity of information on how they spend their money
and a waste of effort on the part of too many of their self-perpet-
uating affiliates. In contrast with business or government, it was
stated, these agencies lack built-in criteria for evaluating expenditure decisions. It was concluded that greater efficiency
has been achieved in fund raising than in spending and that a
reduction in the number of agencies is indicated [66, pp. 30–31].

An implicit assumption is that the amount of money that can
be raised in a locality by volunteers is independent of the number of agencies and causes active in it, that is, that the potential fund for all health causes is a constant; in fact, appeals
may reinforce one another [100, p. 55]. It is implied that lack
of criteria for evaluation represents a peculiar deficiency of
voluntary health agencies, rather than a knotty problem in the
operation of the nonbusiness sectors of the economy. Vickrey
surmises that, owing to personal involvement, voluntary activity
carried out on a small scale is likely to be more efficient than
such activity carried out on a large scale [100, p. 37]. It goes
without saying, of course, that uniform accounting and uniform
reporting of financial data are desirable.

Voluntary Hospitals

Philanthropic income is one of several sources of support
for the voluntary (nonprofit) hospital. Such income has increased in amount but declined in relation to the total. Most of
the percentage decline occurred between 1935 and 1950, and
since then the decline has been small [174, pp. 492–93]. Mean-
while the amount of health insurance benefits has expanded, and
government has assumed greater formal responsibility for financing the care of public charges in hospitals. The result is
that scarcely anybody receives hospital care today without some-
one's paying the hospital for it, at least in part. Free care has,
in effect, become a computed measure of the value of the care
not paid for by, or in behalf of, patients.

Although central fund raising introduces a measure of correction, philanthropic income still is unequally distributed among hospitals and is almost absent in some. In one large city the rate of increase in centrally raised funds has been lagging behind earnings on investments, which among all forms of philanthropic income accrue to the fewest hospitals [174, pp. 439, 454].

There is, moreover, an increasing tendency for certain central fund-raising agencies to distribute money according to arithmetic formula and to avoid discretionary grants to hospitals [174, p. 445]. This has vitiated one of the major advantages attributed to philanthropy, namely, its relative freedom and flexibility of action (100, p. 36].

Catholic hospitals receive almost all the income reported as donated services of Sisters. Such income produces a different effect from philanthropic cash contributions. When the latter appear in a hospital's book of account, they reflect instantaneously an improvement in its financial position. When the former are entered in the books of account, only a potential improvement is recorded. The reason is that an increase in the value of donated services is charged to expenses at the same time that it is credited to income. An improvement in financial position occurs only when steps are taken to convert the higher cost into higher charges to, or in behalf of, patients [174, pp. 450–51]. Such conversion is facilitated when third-party purchasers (insurance plans or government) agree to incorporate the services of Sisters at prevailing salaries in their base of payment.

Most philanthropic income of hospitals is still available for general purposes, including the financing of free care. An increasing tendency toward earmarking gifts for designated purposes, however, does create temptations for hospitals to undertake what can be readily financed rather than what is needed and might be financed only with extra effort. Today it is easier to raise money for construction and research than for service programs or even demonstrations.

It is recognized that earmarked monies have furthered the development of some desirable programs, such as the employment of full-time chiefs of clinical service in hospitals not staffed by medical schools. The disadvantage of earmarked funds lies in the difficulty of maintaining a flexible and balanced program of expenditures over the years.

D. TAX FUNDS, EXEMPTIONS, AND DEDUCTIONS

When government is a source of funds for health and medical services, it may purchase them from others, produce them and provide them without charge or below cost, or subsidize their production in or purchase from the private sector.

Tax funds have traditionally been used to pay for certain public health services furnished in behalf of the entire community and for certain personal health services rendered to members of designated groups. The postwar era has witnessed the addition of grants to assist the construction of nonprofit (voluntary, state, and municipal) hospitals and research facilities and an expansion of expenditures for medical research. Tax funds are not yet employed directly to pay for personal health services for the population at large nor, with minor exceptions, for medical education. The tax laws do, however, provide certain exemptions and deductions that serve to reduce the financial burden of costly illness.

The Amount of Tax Funds

Government's share of total health and medical care expenditures, as officially reported by the Social Security Administration, has fluctuated around one quarter for more than a decade and has shown little or no change in the past six years [21, p. 10]. By making alternative assumptions as to what items of expenditure to count and in which sector of the economy to count them, Davis was able to show that in 1951 the proportion of government to total health and medical care expenditures varied by as much as six percentage points [5, p. 438]. Today the variation due to changes in his assumptions would be smaller, for the relative importance of the items involved has declined in the past decade and some of the concepts employed require modification.

Davis varied three items: (a) military expenditures for

health and medical services; (*b*) construction expenditures by private hospitals (in this context, voluntary plus proprietary) plus depreciation; and (*c*) medical expenditures by certain beneficiaries of government. Their respective amounts in 1951 were $600 million, $470 million, and $600 million, which related to total health and medical care expenditures of $14,200 million (when all expenditures are counted) [5, p. 438].

The military item. For the fiscal year 1961 the military item was officially reported at $0.7 billion [21, p. 10], or 2.5 percent of total health and medical care expenditures of $29.0 billion; this compares with 4.2 percent in 1951. Analysis of detailed data for the fiscal year 1955 by the Hoover Commission indicates that the medical care figure for that year, $603 million (the same as reported by Merriam), is part of a larger total. Accordingly, it seems appropriate to raise the official figure [76, p. 64].

There is a question whether the military item should be counted under health and medical care expenditures. True, the amount spent for health and medical care by the military is heavily affected by the size of the armed forces. However, the amount is not impervious to influences from the civilian economy. In the interest of efficiency an appreciable reduction has been effected in the ratio of physicians to troops, as expanded air transportation was substituted in part for physicians stationed at military bases. Similarly, financial rewards in the civilian economy affect the salary and allowances of physicians in the armed forces. In consequence of changes introduced after World War II, a physician in the military today receives a stipend beyond that paid to officers of the same rank in other branches of the service and a higher initial rank when appointed.

To analyze problems pertaining to the use of resources in the health field, it is necessary, in the writer's judgment, to take cognizance of the health and medical care expenditures incurred by the military. In preparing trend data on the role of government in the civilian economy, it may be preferable to exclude the item. Both purposes can be served by showing the item separately.

Construction expenditures and depreciation. Expenditures

for hospital construction were originally regarded as an equivalent for current charges on capital [61, p. 8]. Included in such charges are depreciation, interest on debt, and interest on the equity invested in physical plant.

Expenditures for construction are a reasonable approximation of capital charges when the quantity of physical plant is constant, but not when it is expanding. The continuing rise in the cost of construction is another source of overstatement, for depreciation on the existing stock of capital, valued at historical cost, would be a lower figure.

Depreciation on capital is one of the elements of gross national product (GNP). When health and medical care expenditures are related to GNP, they should include an allowance for depreciation. When related to net national product (NNP), they should not.

It appears, therefore, that it was a mistake for the President's Commission on the Health Needs of the Nation to include expenditures for hospital construction in the numerator when it related health and medical care expenditures to NNP [29, Vol. 4, p. 151]. Similarly, Davis was mistaken in counting both private expenditures for hospital construction and depreciation when he related health and medical care expenditures to GNP [5, pp. 313, 438]; for this is double counting. (Nor is Davis altogether consistent. He counts expenditures for construction of public hospitals and excludes their depreciation. The stated reason, that replacement of public hospitals is financed from current tax receipts [5, p. 439], is not valid, although it fortuitously leads to the correct procedure.)

In measuring the amount of health and medical care expenditures, it is easier to take account of construction expenditures and to neglect depreciation. Not only is there a lack of information on the amount of depreciation of equipment in the offices of physicians and dentists, but there is no information on the extent to which depreciation expense is reflected in the published statistics on expenditures for hospital care [174, p. 480]. In view of the increasing willingness of insurance plans and government agencies to pay for depreciation, especially if the payment is set aside (funded) for capital purposes, it is reasonable to suppose that more hospitals are entering larger depreciation charges on their books and that the amount of depreciation embodied in reported hospital expenditures is rising. (A rough estimate of the current amount is of the order of $0.1 billion [76, Table 10].)

Expenditures by public assistance recipients. Davis's data on medical care expenditures out of public assistance grants and noncontributory pensions derive from Harris, who noted that certain medical care expenditures are incurred privately but are in fact financed by government. Counting all income maintenance programs, other than benefits under social security (then the Old Age and Survivors Insurance Program), he had estimated the sum involved at $600–$650 million in the fiscal year 1949–50 [68, p. 4]. Logically, one could argue that today the bulk of social security benefits also derive from tax funds and not from employer and employee contributions. However, if the criterion for assigning an item to a particular sector is who authorizes the amounts and the types of expenditure, medical care expenditures financed from social security benefits belong in the private sector. Following this line of reasoning, medical care expenditures financed by other types of pension also belong in the private sector so long as the amount of pension is not affected by the size of the medical care bill. This holds true even when the pension is not earned through prior contributions.

Today most medical care expenditures in behalf of public assistance recipients are paid directly to the providers of services. In 1961 the amount of vendor payments was $0.6 billion [21, p. 10]. A much smaller amount, of the order of $0.2 billion, was spent by the recipients of care, subject to reimbursement from welfare agencies [76, Table 10]. The latter amount should be transferred from the private to the public sector, on the ground that public officials authorize the amount spent and have it added to the relief recipient's grant. Robertson would go further and effect the transfer even in the absence of specific augmentation [88, pp. 31–32].

In addition to the above, the major adjustment in the public sector is the removal of most workmen's compensation benefits (see Chapter III, Section A). The net outcome of the several adjustments, the writer has found, is to leave unchanged the official figure on the size of the public sector. For 1961 it amounts to 24 percent of total health and medical care expenditures. The appreciable changes wrought by the rearrangements and adjustments are in the business and the philanthropic sectors, on the one hand, and in the consumer sector, on the other hand, with the former two being larger than officially reported and the latter smaller. In addition, the federal government gains at the expense of state and local governments [76, Table 3].

Exemptions and Deductions

Government pays indirectly for a part of private expenditures for medical care through the medical care deduction allowed under the individual income tax [68, p. 4]; this will be discussed below. Losses in government revenues also accrue through the deduction of philanthropic contributions to health causes and the exemption of nonprofit hospitals from the real property tax. These two items are probably intended as incentives to promote the provision of services through the voluntary (nonprofit) form of organization.

Philanthropic contributions to health agencies derive from many sources, including living persons, corporations, foundations, religious organizations, and bequests, all of which are subject to different tax laws [73, p. 221]. A rough estimate of the tax loss due to such contributions would be of the order of $0.3 billion, or somewhere between one third and one half of the total amount claimed as deductions.

For some purposes, such as a comparison of cost between home care and hospital care, it is important to take account of the value of the real estate tax exemption, which would constitute an addition to the reported figures on health and medical care expenditures. (This applies to government hospitals as well. The rate of the real property tax would presumably be lower if the tax base were enlarged, but this effect is perhaps of a secondary order of magnitude.) The writer has estimated the value of the exemption of hospitals from the real property tax and from water charges in one large city. It approximates 5 percent of reported hospital cost [174, pp. 483, 488]. Perhaps the figure would be lower for the country as a whole, for real estate values and tax rates are lower in small cities and in rural areas; an estimate of $0.4 billion for the nation is not unreasonable.

One of the most important contributions by government—direct or indirect—to the financing of personal health services is the cost to the federal treasury of the medical expense deduction under the individual income tax. For the year 1951 Harris estimated the value of private medical care expenditures with public funds from this source at $500 million [68, p. 8]; this figure was probably too high. In 1956 Kahn estimated the amount at $700 million [73, p. 137]. For 1960 the value of the medical care deduction to taxpayers is estimated at $1 billion [76, p. 54]. An additional $375 million is lost by the Treasury owing to medical expenses included in the tax returns of income recipients who take the standard deduction; it is reasonable to assume that in the absence of a medical expense deduction the standard deduction would be lower than at present.

Revenue losses under state income taxes are not considered in the above estimates.

It is believed appropriate to retain the tax value of the medical expense deduction in the private sector for most purposes, since the decisions governing the expenditures are made here [102, p. 370]. The item, however, might be taken into account in comparing the relative costs of alternative governmental programs.

The medical care deduction in the federal income tax was enacted in 1942. The Treasury's intention was to help defray "extraordinary" medical expenses in excess of a specified percentage of a family's net income [72, p. 395; 73, p. 127]. For fear of possible abuses a ceiling was imposed. Subsequently both the floor and the ceiling were liberalized, and for persons 65 years and over the floor was removed.

The floor is an arbitrary figure [83, p. 307]. In 1953 the median proportion of family medical care expenditures to income was 4.1 percent. The floor of 5 percent then prevailing seems consistent with the basic rationale of the deduction [72,

p. 396]. In 1958 the median figure of family medical care expenditures to income was closer to 5 percent, the mean having risen from 4.8 to 5.5 percent [53, p. 18]. Accordingly, the current floor of 3–4 percent, depending on one's expenditures for drugs, appears to be on the low side. Nevertheless, there are those who would further reduce it [65, p. 145].

Consistent with the Treasury's intention is the view that the medical care deduction is a device to refine tax paying ability [102, pp. 369–70]. A family burdened with heavy medical charges is deemed less able to pay taxes than a family of similar composition with the same income that does not incur such charges [2, p. 267]. If the deduction were intended primarily as an incentive to taxpayers to do certain things in furtherance of social objectives, a tax credit (a subtraction from computed tax liability) might be more appropriate [73, p. 128].

The income tax deduction may be viewed as quasi-insurance. The premium takes the form of a higher rate of tax paid by those who do not incur sufficient medical care expenditures to receive the deduction. The benefit is the reduction in tax due to the deduction when expenditures are large. However, purchasers of voluntary health insurance reduce the annual fluctuations in their medical care expenditures and, accordingly, receive smaller benefits from the income tax deduction than persons who do not buy insurance. The uninsured are thereby subsidized [72, p. 398]. Kahn noted a possible offset in the tendency of insured persons to incur larger expenditures for medical care than their uninsured counterparts [73, p. 135].

Public finance specialists view personal deductions under the individual income tax with skepticism and would limit them to the greatest extent possible. However, they accept and some even favor the medical expense deduction, because of the unpredictable and often involuntary character of medical care expenditures [34, p. 148]. Large expenditures for medical care are not elements in a higher standard of living but are associated with the misfortunes of illness. Some would moderate the impact of the deduction on government revenues, by raising the floor below which the medical care deduction is not operative [72, p. 396] or by changing the Treasury's participation from a deduction from the tax base to a tax credit against a stated fraction of expenditures [102, p. 370]. The latter has also been proposed as a device to stimulate voluntary health insurance [65, p. 145].

E. SELECTED GOVERNMENT PROGRAMS

There is a traditional division of responsibility for health and medical services among the federal government, the states, and local governments. The United States finances care for the military and some of their dependents, for veterans to varying degrees, for merchant seamen, and for Indians. Including grants-in-aid to the states, the federal government accounts for almost one half of total government expenditures, or one eighth of all expenditures for health and medical care [76, Table 3]. With military expenditures excluded, the federal government's shares are at 42 and 10 percent, respectively. Almost all tax funds in medical research are federal, as are the grants by government toward the construction of voluntary (nonprofit) hospitals.

The states have major responsibility for mental hospitals (operating four fifths of all beds) and share with local governments the responsibility in caring for patients with tuberculosis and in financing personal health and medical services for public assistance recipients and the medically indigent. Medical care for four categories of public assistance (aid to the blind, aid to families with dependent children, old age assistance, and aid to the permanently and totally disabled), as well as for the recipients of medical care for the aged, is partly reimbursed by the federal government. The division of the financial burden between the state government and local units of government varies among the states and is affected by provisions for state aid and tax sharing under programs other than health and medical care.

Federal Programs

Medical research. The first substantial federal appropriation for medical research was voted in 1918. A permanent program was initiated in 1937 with the establishment of the National

Cancer Institute [87, p. 28]. The most rapidly expanding public expenditures in the health field in the postwar period are for medical research. Between 1947 and 1960 appropriations to the National Institutes of Health increased 20 to 30 percent annually [87, p. 40]. Federal support has become an increasingly important component of a growing total. Between 1951 and 1963 total expenditures increased more than 9 times, from $163 million to $1,550 million, while the federal share rose 13 times, from $73 million to $973 million [76, p. 47].

Three fourths of the federal medical research funds are spent in facilities outside the government—at universities and institutes—and are distributed under the guidance of a network of advisory committees and councils whose members are drawn from the scientific community. The principal vehicle of expenditure has been the project research grant to an investigator in response to a detailed and specific application for research support. A movement has begun, however, toward larger and longer-term grants for more generally stated purposes. The needs of research have also led to the substantial support of teaching programs in the health sciences [87, pp. 51, 88].

Veterans. The largest of the federal medical care programs is that for veterans. Almost all care is furnished in the Veterans Administration's own hospitals, and very little is purchased.

Operation of hospitals by government probably has an effect on the amount of tax funds spent. Criteria of eligibility for admission are likely to be more liberal in the government's own hospitals, in which overhead is paid for and an empty bed is an obvious waste, than in hospitals operated by others, from which care is purchased patient day by patient day. When public facilities exist, the line of demarcation between those who do and do not receive care at public expense is not so sharp [222, p. 39].

The Veterans Administration hospitals care for veterans with service connected disabilities and, in accordance with a specified priority scheme, for as many veterans with nonservice connected diseases and injuries as can be accommodated. Critics assert that the program of hospital care for veterans fails to reflect a consistent and rational policy for discharging government's responsibility to the veterans. Yet, it would seem that, insofar as Congress appropriates money for the construction of facilities and then appropriates money for their operation, it is in fact defining the size and scope of program. One would think that a given amount of money could be equated with the operation of a certain number of beds. Toward the close of the Eisenhower administration the implicit policy on the size of the Veterans Administration system was confirmed when a ceiling of 125,000 hospital beds was established. Since then nursing home facilities have become the object of attention.

A census taken in June, 1957, furnished information for the first time on the role of the Veterans Administration in providing hospital care to the nation's veterans. Of 188,000 veterans in the hospital on a given day, 110,000 were receiving care under Veterans Administration auspices and 78,000 under other auspices, 58 and 42 percent, respectively [98, p. I-2]. In terms of the number of patients annually admitted to the hospital the role of the Veterans Administration hospitals is smaller, namely, one fifth [45, p. 28]. It follows that Veterans Administration institutions care for a large proportion of the veterans hospitalized for long stays.

In 1949 Ginzberg pointed out that psychiatric and tuberculosis patients are usually public charges and that patients with other long-term illness (defined as a stay of thirty or more days in the hospital) frequently are. From a financial standpoint, he concluded, only 8 percent of all patient days in the Veterans Administration hospitals might possibly be transferable to community hospitals [64c, p. 45]. The principal issue, as he saw it, is the financial relations between the federal and state (and local) governments and not competition between government and the private sector.

Military dependents. A vital consideration in formulating a policy for the care of dependents of the military is to secure a variety of patients for the military hospitals. Availability of diverse clinical material is essential for medical education and for recruiting and retaining medical staff. The idea of paying civilian hospitals for the care of dependents stems from a desire to raise the rate of military re-enlistments through improved morale and by extending more equitable treatment to dependents who live at a distance from military posts. The size of the program has varied with fluctuations in the amount of annual appropriations; in turn, these have required changes in the criteria governing eligibility for care.

Under this program the federal government pays hospitals and physicians through the instrumentality of health insurance plans. Following negotiations, the Blue Cross Association was chosen as the fiscal intermediary in two regions of the country (East Coast and West Coast) and a representative of the commercial insurance industry as the intermediary in the third region (Midwest). The federal government reimburses the plans for payments to the providers of services and adds an allowance for administrative expenses. Benefits do not cover all expenses, and the patient pays a specified amount, a so-called deductible.

It should be noted that there is no element of insurance in this program, though insurance would not be precluded by the characteristics of the population. This is a significant difference between the dependents' medical care program and the much larger public programs for the medically indigent that are administered at the state and local levels (see below).

Vocational rehabilitation. In discussions of the newer categories of persons whose medical care is financed through tax funds the language of economic cost and benefit often appears. A good illustration of such a category is vocational rehabilitation. Advocates of an expanded program point to lower relief payments and higher tax revenues, as well as to enlarged output. Questions regarding the validity of the arithmetic are raised in Chapter VII, Section B.

Substantial increases in the clientele of the program were originally projected, but these have not materialized. The statistical base was inadequate to support the projection of patient load. In addition, success in rehabilitation is usually associated with a high degree of clinical selectivity by the physician specialist (physiatrist). The results achieved under favorable circumstances may not be applicable to the disabled population at large or to a disabled population with certain (social, cultural, and so forth) disadvantages.

State and Local Programs

Insurers and fiscal agents. State and local government agencies seldom employ the health insurance mechanism to pay for the care of the sick poor. The reasons differ for the medically indigent and the indigent (recipients of public assistance).

A medically indigent person is one who cannot afford to pay for the cost of a given illness, although he can pay for his normal living expenses. He is identified as medically indigent after becoming ill. Once ill, he is, of course, not eligible to buy insurance. For a group to be insurable its members must share some common characteristic prior to illness, such as income, occupation, employment status, and so forth.

Since recipients of public assistance are identified prior to illness, they are not precluded from insurance. However, certain groups, particularly the aged, use more services than the rest of the population and would constitute a drain on any voluntary insurance plan aimed at, and paid by, the employed segment of the population. Even so, recipients of Old Age Assistance are reported to be insured for physicians' services in five states and for hospital care in one state. Use of the insurance mechanism more frequently to meet the cost of physicians' services than of hospital services may reflect the fact that differences in utilization between the aged and the population at large are not so great for the former services. In three states Blue Shield (for physicians' services) is employed as fiscal agent, not as insurer, and in four states Blue Cross (for hospital services) serves as fiscal agent [97, pp. 125–26]. In some states the official welfare agency is reluctant to pay through an intermediary, because it can buy the same services directly at lower fees.

Hospital care. Of the state and local tax funds that finance short-term hospital care, 30 percent purchase services from voluntary hospitals [174, p. 510]. The terms of purchase vary a great deal. The government agency may be stringent in certifying (approving) patients for payment and limit them to emergency admissions. At the opposite pole, government may approve patients in voluntary hospitals for payment under the same criteria as in its own hospitals. Either policy on the certification of patients may be associated with a high, moderate, or low daily rate of payment.

The policy most likely to appeal to hospitals, and therefore to be adopted by government, is a rate calculated on the basis of individual hospital cost. Criteria for certifying patients appear to be of secondary interest. Implicit is the assumption that there is no connection between the daily rate of payment and the number of patients government will pay for, so that the hospitals' income from tax funds is, in effect, determined exclusively by the rate of payment.

Almost all long-term care paid for by state and local tax funds is provided in government hospitals [76, Table 11]. This has been historically true of psychiatric services, which are concentrated in state hospitals, and of tuberculosis services, which are distributed between the states and municipalities (counties and cities). Only with the expansion of proprietary nursing homes in the 1950s did the purchase of long-term care with tax funds come to the fore.

Impact of Additional Funds

Availability of funds can—and does—influence the scope and direction of program development. For example, money for crippled children has contributed to the establishment of comprehensive programs of care for premature infants, for children with heart disease, and so forth. Amendments to the Social Security Act furnished the basis for the expansion of proprietary nursing homes and led to the conversion of some county homes for the aged into infirmaries for the sick [174, pp. 407–8].

Sometimes, however, the effect of the new money is nullified if it serves to replace existing money. An example of the substitution of federal for state and local funds may be found in the working of the program of Medical Assistance for the Aged (Kerr-Mills program) in some states. In one large city (New York City) new state money for community mental health programs was applied largely to reduce the City's expenditures in the psychiatric services of its own hospitals.

Even where additional monies are voted, they may not achieve the stated aims [25, p. 11]. For example, funds alone have not enabled existing public home infirmaries (nursing home units in municipal general hospitals) to achieve proper staffing nor led to the construction of more of them, an objective espoused by many students of long-term care. Other factors, such as lack of interest (and perhaps also of ability) to care for the aged and opposition by medical school faculties to staffing long-term facilities, have been decisive [172, pp. 22, 52].

IV. SUPPLY OF PERSONNEL

It is helpful to introduce a discussion of the supply of health personnel with a brief discussion of the general nature of supply in economics.

A. WHAT IS SUPPLY?

Supply is a schedule, not a single point. A supply schedule lists the alternative prices at which various quantities of a good or a service will be offered at a given time (more accurately, over an interval). It represents the forces impinging on price and output from the production side, so that usually (under competitive market conditions and when there is time for production to take place, in contrast to a situation in which sales are drawn exclusively from inventory) a supply curve (the graphical representation of a supply schedule) derives from (when it is not identical with) a particular cost curve [43a, p. 147]. Movements along the supply curve show the variation between the quantities of a good (or a service) offered and prices, on the assumption that certain other things are held constant. The other things are technical knowledge or the state of the arts (the economist's production function); the prices of other things that are closely related in production; and the supply curves of the factors of production (labor, capital, and so forth).

To hold other things constant is not to neglect them. Rather, when one of the other things changes, the supply curve shifts upward (or downward), so that at a given price smaller (larger) quantities of the good or service are offered.

Time is neither instantaneous nor geared to the calendar. The notion of time in the supply of economic goods, which stems from Alfred Marshall, pertains to the problem at hand and has to do with the adjustments that a firm or an industry can effect in combining inputs of the several factors of production. In the long run a firm can make all necessary adjustments in the scale of operations, including that of entering or leaving the industry. In the short run the size of plant is fixed, and output can be varied only by changing certain inputs of labor and materials. A long-run supply curve for a given quantity of output is flatter in shape (more elastic) than the short-run curve, owing chiefly to the different shapes of the supply curves of the factors of production to the industry.

The supply of hospital service can be analyzed in conventional terms by inquiring into the shapes of the short-term and long-term marginal cost curves and into the reasons that shifts in these curves (and in the associated average cost curves) occur. When costs to the firm or to an industry are of central concern, the demand for factor inputs is said to be a derived demand and is not the focus of attention. Although conceptually the analysis of supply and demand conditions is the same for a product as for a factor of production, there are sufficient differences in substance to warrant separate treatment of the two markets.

However, in the case of physicians' services it would seem artificial to analyze the market for the product separately from the market for physicians. The reasons are two-fold: on the demand side the consumer is heavily influenced by his physician in the quantities of services taken, so that the demand can be said to be for a physician; and, more important, on the supply side the quantity of services the profession is ready to offer depends largely on the number of physicians in practice and but little on the prices that can be charged per unit of service rendered [124, p. 155].

Accordingly, the supply of physician services and of hospital services will be treated differently and separately. As for other health personnel, dentists are usually dealt with in comparison with physicians; they do not receive separate treatment here.

In a study of nurses it is important to distinguish between those employed by hospitals and all others; a comprehensive study of the economic status of the former is currently in progress at Washington University, St. Louis [150]. An earlier study of nurses and their function has been superseded by events [115], in that the recommended substitution of practical nurses and nurses' aides for some registered nurses is no longer at issue. The writer's analysis of hospital nurses in one large city compared staffing ratios in two hospital systems (voluntary and municipal) and devoted special attention to the roles of private duty nurses and student nurses [174, pp. 237–41]. (See Chapters IV, Section D, and V, Section B.)

Strictly speaking, the concept of a supply curve is not applicable to drugs, since the number of firms producing a given drug is small and these firms are not willing to offer various quantities of drugs at alternative prices. The firms' decisions on price and output are influenced by the effect of the quantity taken on price (the difference between average revenue, that is, price, and marginal revenue), which depends on the shape of each firm's demand curve. There is reason to expect that an analysis of the economics of the drug industry would yield a substantial pay-off.

Chapters on personnel (mostly physicians) and on facilities (mostly hospitals) are followed by a chapter on the problems of organization and coordination in the health and medical care industry.

B. THE RELATIVE SUPPLY OF LABOR TO TWO OCCUPATIONS

Discussion of the supply of physicians will be facilitated by a brief introduction on the factors that determine the supply of labor to particular occupations. It is convenient to follow Friedman in employing a relative supply curve for two occupations at a time (the relative number of man-hours supplied varying with relative wage rates) [11, p. 213]. Although these remarks apply to any two occupations, there is no harm in thinking of the one as physicians and the other as dentists.

The factors that determine the supply of labor to a particular occupation are largely independent of the factors that determine the total supply of labor to an economy [11, p. 211]. If all individuals had the same abilities and made identical evaluations of the relative merits of two occupations, the relative supply curve would be perfectly elastic (horizontal). The level of wages would be determined exclusively by those conditions of supply that make the two occupations equal attractive financially, such as seasonal and cyclical fluctuations in employment, length of training, direct cost of training, length of working life in an occupation, the pattern of earnings over a lifetime, and so on [43b, pp. 196–97]. Conditions of demand alone would determine the number of workers in each occupation. Conversely, the supply curve would be perfectly inelastic (vertical) if some persons held an absolute preference for occupation A over occupation B while others similarly preferred B over A, regardless of financial returns. In actuality, differences among individuals in ability and in tastes lead to differences in the relative wage rates regarded as making two occupations equally attractive. In consequence, the supply curve has a positive slope [11, pp. 219–20].

Friedman classifies the factors affecting the supply curve of labor in an occupation into three categories: (a) those that determine the relative pecuniary attractiveness of occupations; (b) variability of income; and (c) nonpecuniary differences among occupations. The second and third categories comprise the factors that reflect the peculiar characteristics of the supply of labor noted by Marshall. Thus, the worker sells his work but retains capital ownership in himself; the seller of labor must deliver it personally, making a tie-in contract between the sale of his labor power and the "purchase" of the conditions of work [11, pp. 212–14].

A given supply curve relates the relative numbers of persons and relative incomes, on the assumption that other things are given. Among these things are peoples' attitudes toward the variability of income and the attractiveness of occupations to them, in terms of the conditions of work, prestige, location, and so forth. A broad consensus about the other things serves to shift the supply curve upward or downward, the extent of the shift measuring the price people are willing to pay (or require to be paid to them) for nonpecuniary advantages (or disadvantages) [11, pp. 218–19].

Similarly, a rise in productivity may be viewed as a downward shift in the supply curve. However, treatment of the length of the work week is more problematical, for it involves both income and substitution effects, and changes in hours may be described by a "backward bending" supply curve of labor. (When an increase in demand occurs and wages rise, the substitution effect makes leisure more expensive and tends to increase the number of hours worked. The rise in wages also increases real income and leads the worker to buy more of various goods, including leisure, thereby reducing the number of hours worked.) Under given circumstances there is no way to determine the outcome without empirical study [34, pp. 151–52].

Differences in wage rates (incomes) among occupations depend then on differences in financial return and in cost and on differences in tastes. They also depend on the level of demand, large or small. These are so-called equalizing differences. In addition there are differences in wage rates due to the existence of noncompeting groups, that is, barriers to the free choice of occupation; and there are transitional differences, due to lags in adjustment to changes in demand or supply [11, pp. 212–13].

C. THE SUPPLY OF PHYSICIANS

In discussing health manpower there is a tendency to concentrate on physicians. One reason is that physicians activate almost all other health personnel, including nurses and pharmacists. In comparison with dentists, their realm is larger—the entire human body—and their graduate education takes longer and is more arduous. Physicians are called members of the health team, but their preeminence as its leaders is unchallenged, whether the task is patient care, research, planning, or administration.

Supply curves for physicians differ in slope over time, being more elastic in the long run. In the short run the supply curve is quite inelastic, since the number of physicians is substantially independent of prevailing income [124, p. 155]. In the long run the supply curve is likely to be positively sloped. Although the number of physicians who withdraw from the occupation because of death is independent of economic factors, the number seeking to enter—the number of applicants to medical school—is probably influenced, among other factors, by pecuniary prospects, that is, by the average (arithmetic mean) income individuals expect to receive [124, p. 156]. (It has been suggested, however, that the number of applicants to medical school is determined by nonmarket forces [55, p. 953].)

Since few physicians announce retirement from practice, some retired physicians and larger numbers of semiactive physicians remain in the count of practitioners. According to one rule of thumb, the number of physicians aged sixty-five and over are convertible into full-time active equivalents at a ratio of one third [114, p. 317].

Physicians trained abroad—both American citizens and permanent immigrants—constituted an appreciable and increasing source of supply during the 1950s. Nevertheless, American medical schools continue as the chief source by far, having contributed more than 90 percent of all licensed physicians in this country. Between 1940 and 1960 the number of their graduates rose by 40 percent.

Unlike most other types of professional school, American medical schools continue to reject large numbers of qualified applicants. However, the number of applicants has declined since the early postwar peak. For some years the downward trend continued both absolutely and in relation to the total number of college graduates, but a reversal in absolute numbers has occurred. Since the number of openings in medical school has increased, the chances of admission per applicant have improved from one of three to better than one of two.

Medical educators view developments in the 1950s with alarm, mainly on the ground that the quality of the candidates has been impaired. Trend data for the past decade on college grades and admission test scores do not substantiate these fears. Rather there is reason to believe that medicine is facing competition from the glamorous basic sciences for the top 5 percent or so of the talent pool. In this competition medicine may be at a disadvantage, since it requires a longer training period before an appreciable income is earned and the schools offer fewer scholarships [133, p. 20].

A more serious threat to the quality of physicians is posed by the restrictive admission practices of some of the state-owned medical schools. Since out of state residents are barred, available spaces are sometimes filled by state residents with poor academic records [139, p. 239]. Limiting admissions to residents is intended to help assure an adequate supply of practicing physicians in a state. The admission of nonresidents is seen as a subsidy to persons who are likely to practice elsewhere.

The writer believes that this justification may be erroneous. Intern and residency training takes place in a nation-wide network of hospitals, and the site of graduate education is a more potent influence on the location of a physician's practice than the site of his medical school. In public medical schools 82 percent of the students are drawn from the home state, compared with 48 percent in private schools. However, only 55 percent of the graduates of public medical schools practice in the same state, compared with 38 percent of the graduates of private schools. The former incur a loss of 26 percentage points and the latter 10 percentage points [147, p. 1,091].

Moreover, unlike dentists, American-educated physicians encounter few professional barriers in relocating their practice from one state to another. Not only are some salaried positions exempt from the requirement of a state license, but in many circumstances a license can readily be obtained by reciprocity or endorsement, without formal examination [128, p. 7]. (Unlike dentistry and law, there is no correlation in medicine between failure rates among applicants for licensure by examination and average state practitioners' incomes [128, p. 19].) The uncertainties surrounding the acquisition of a hospital staff appointment in a new city constitute a more serious barrier to moving, particularly for a specialist who earns a good part of his living in the hospital.

In considering the availability of physicians to render health and medical care it is necessary to take cognizance of three additional factors: (a) length of the work week; (b) productivity; and (c) the performance of functions other than patient care.

The average time available to render services depends on the work week, the proportion of time allotted to medical education and research, attendance at professional meetings, and length of vacation. Although a physician's participation in teaching and research has certain economic ramifications—greater prestige (hence, higher fees), more referrals, and increased productivity as a result of self-improvement and through assistance from the house staff in caring for hospitalized patients—it is preponderantly a nonpecuniary phenomenon, a matter of professional obligation and status. Some of the other factors are, however, essentially economic phenomena, being heavily influenced by the physician's fees and income. There is a wide range to the number of hours a physician can be expected to devote to patient care—from 2,000 hours a year to 1,440 and 1,200 [139, p. 226].

The productivity of physicians (defined in terms of the number of visits by patients) has obviously increased in the past generation or two, with the widespread adoption of the telephone, the speeding up of travel, the transfer of the bulk of patient care from the home to the doctor's office and the hospital, and the increased employment of auxiliary hospital personnel, both in traditional categories, such as that of nurses, and in new ones, such as that of technicians. Only the rate of increase in productivity is a moot question (see Chapter VII, Section A), especially in comparison with the rate of increase in the demand for physicians' services.

There is, on the other hand, an increasing tendency for physicians to perform activities other than patient care. Activities that claim their attention are medical education, medical research, public health, hospital administration, and so on. The presence of full-time teachers in medical schools and their hospitals is a sequel to the Flexner Report on medical education, and the presence of full-time physicians in nonuniversity hospitals is a more recent, postwar development, which accelerated in the 1950s.

D. IMPLICATIONS OF SPECIALIZATION

Medicine resembles other professions in moving toward increasing specialization, for available knowledge is too voluminous for one person to master. The rapid growth of specialization among physicians creates problems for the public and the profession.

Effect on Practice

Medical care was formerly furnished by the general practitioner, the family physician. There were few occasions to coordinate services, since referral of a patient to a consultant for diagnosis and advice on therapy was a rare event. Today continuity of care is still regarded as the touchstone of good medicine, but a single practitioner can no longer be expected to provide all necessary services. Specialization implies a division of labor, and a visit to the specialist is a frequent occurrence.

One difficulty with the notion that the general physician will play the role of coordinator of medical care for the family is that the number of general practitioners is declining, not only as a proportion of the total number of physicians but also numerically. The decline was accelerated by the transformation of specialty training from a prolonged apprenticeship of an active practitioner into a formal, almost academic, residency program. Today few physicians who intend to specialize take time between the internship and residency to engage in general practice. Although there are certain fields in which a gradual transition takes place in the course of practice, such as from obstetrics to gynecology, there is still no pause for general practice.

The supply of labor to a particular medical specialty is more elastic than to the profession as a whole, for there is greater mobility within medicine than between medicine and other occupations [43*b*, p. 201]. However, formalization of training requirements and the choice of a specialty early in a physician's career serve to reduce mobility among fields of specialization and to make the several supply curves less elastic. As a consequence, one would expect nonequalizing differences in income among specialties to persist longer than formerly [11, p. 219].

Intensive specialization is almost bound to raise the cost of medical services. The specialist feels compelled to perform a thorough examination in his own field. Since he is insecure outside this narrow field, he must refer the patient to another specialist when in doubt. Another source of higher cost is the need to compensate the physician for the postponement of earnings during prolonged training and for whatever lag in income occurs during the early stages of his career as a limited specialist [155, Chapter 2, pp. 9-11]. Still another is the differentiation of product attendant upon specialization and the consequent ability of the physician to influence fees [124, p. 138].

Although less documentation exists on the scope of specialization in the other health professions, the contrast with medicine is so striking as to warrant comment. Equally marked is the contrasting trend in hospitals.

In dentistry the proportion of specialists is small. The route to specialization is still via general practice, the cultivation of a special interest, and the pursuit of postgraduate courses while continuing in practice.

The explanation for the different patterns in medicine and in dentistry is not obvious. One factor undoubtedly is the smaller volume of knowledge to be mastered in dentistry. In a sense, every dentist is already a medical specialist, and further specialization may diminish his interest. Another factor may be the more discretionary character of consumer spending for dental care and the (almost complete) absence of health insurance. It may be that current expenditures for dental care would not support an elaborate structure of specialization. There is also the absence of the hospital as a central force. Finally, the existing situation may represent a time lag.

There is some degree of specialization in nursing, mostly between public health nursing and institutional nursing. The additional time required to prepare for specialization is relatively short, a year or so. Industrial nursing is a specialty akin to public health, but private duty nursing has become to a considerable extent a different, more flexible way of working in an institution [174, p. 240].

Within the hospital nurses specialize on the basis of experience and performance, but boundaries are not rigid. The important difference among nurses is not in the field of specialization but in the level of administrative responsibility. Traditionally, promotion takes place on the administrative ladder, for clinical nursing carries a narrow salary range [115, pp. 85–86]. With the widespread employment of part-time nurses and auxiliary workers, the premium placed on managerial ability is greater than formerly [174, p. 224].

At the same time the role of the specialty hospital has declined. The current emphasis is on making the general hospital more general, by encompassing all or most of the services formerly provided in specialty institutions.

Effect on Graduate Medical Education

The growth of specialization in medicine is intimately associated with the expansion of graduate medical education in hospitals, almost all of which has occurred since 1900. The year 1935 is sometimes cited as the starting point for the present pattern of graduate medical education in this country [174, p. 167].

World War II and its aftermath brought a rapid transformation. In intern training there were two simultaneous developments: (a) the total number of positions offered continued to increase; and (b) the number of positions with a two-year term declined from 25 percent of the total in 1940 to 10 percent in 1949 and to less than 1 percent in 1958. Despite the fact that the number of graduates from American medical schools continued to increase, it was not possible to fill all positions.

The armed forces furnished an impetus to residency training by giving consideration to a physician's diplomate status in classifying and assigning him. After the war many discharged physicians sought residencies for refresher training or in preparation for a specialist's career.

Factors in increased demand for house staff. Both the number of hospitals in this country with approved training programs and the average number of physicians per hospital house staff have increased to the point that the total number of physicians training in hospitals (including graduates of foreign schools) exceeds the number of students in American medical schools. Among the contributing factors are the following [174, pp. 169–70]:

(a) Reduction in the average duration of patient stay in the hospital. A higher proportion of house staff time than formerly is, therefore, spent on the patient's initial examination (medical history and physical examination).

(b) Increasing reliance by attending staff on interns and residents to render medical services to their hospitalized private patients. These services are a major source of increased output— and of higher income—for the private practitioner outside the hospital.

(c) Proliferation of medical specialties and subspecialties, which is accompanied by the desire of hospitals and medical staffs to assign residents to as many services as possible.

(d) A requirement by most specialty boards that a year's training in internal medicine and general surgery, the mother specialties, precede and augment training in the subspecialties.

(e) A rise in the number and proportion of interns and residents who are married and have children. Fewer young physicians are as available as formerly for duty round-the-clock seven days a week.

(f) Finally, and important, the low cost of house staff to the hospital relative to the expected gain for all concerned.

Factors in increased supply of house staff. Expansion of graduate medical education was achieved through (a) an increase in the number of physicians graduated from American medical schools, as previously noted; (b) prolongation of the average duration of graduate medical education; and (c) an influx of physicians from abroad in quest of hospital training in this country.

With the rise in the number and proportion of physicians in specialty practice, the average duration of graduate medical education (internship plus residency) lengthened from an estimated two years in 1940 to 3.5 years in 1956 [107, p. 9; 174, pp. 215-16]. The entire increase occurred in residency training (indeed, the average duration of the internship declined from 15 to 12 months), and most of it is attributable to the increased proportion of physicians who prepare for limited specialized practice rather than to prolongation in the average training time for a given type of practitioner [147, p. 1,092].

The number of foreign-educated physicians serving as house staff in this country rose appreciably in the 1950s. The principal factor was the official exchange program for temporary visitors, which became effective in July, 1949.

Postponement of income. Traditionally interns and residents have served hospitals as a form of cheap labor. Accordingly, their services have been consistently undervalued from the standpoint of the economic allocation of resources [104, pp. 19-20]. It was not until the wartime shortage of civilian physicians that interns were removed from the emergency ambulance service operated by hospitals and lay attendants with training in first aid substituted.

Going without earnings during graduate training accounts for a good part of the differential in average earnings between practicing physicians and those in other occupations [43b, pp. 195-96]. This is not surprising, since the foregoing of income is a major element in the cost of training for any profession. It has been well said, "Medical training is long and costly and, while the ultimate rewards may be sweet, they are discouragingly slow to materialize" [9, p. 338]. Feeling exploited and deprived of a living wage for too long, the young physician may try to recoup promptly upon entry into practice and will succeed in doing so if the demand conditions for physicians' services are favorable.

The income postponement effect resulting from the shift from apprenticeship to residency training has, perhaps, been cushioned to some extent. In the past there was considerable idle time in the initial phase of a specialty career while referrals were building up [136, p. 47]. Today the lag in initial earnings by young practitioners is shorter [42, p. 205]. Upon completing his residency, the young physician often can obtain remunerative employment, temporary and part-time, with insurance companies and industrial concerns or can increase his earnings in private practice by serving as a substitute for an established physician nights and weekends.

Characteristics of the labor market. A recent study of the intern market concluded that it possesses some of the characteristics of a competitive market. Thus, the numbers of sellers and buyers are large; entry into the market is controlled but not unduly restrictive; information is adequate on both sides; and the trend is toward payment in salary rather than in kind [104, pp. 4–9]. On the other hand, some of the market's characteristics point to noncompetitive behavior. Among them are the presence of price discrimination (higher stipends for married physicians); persistent price uniformity in a geographic area, which is sometimes taken as evidence of collusion; and the importance of an institution's prestige in attracting recruits [104, pp. 21–25].

It should be noted that uniformity of stipends need not be evidence of collusion. At a given location the number of buyers (hospitals) may be small, and the sellers (young physicians) may prefer to train there in order to test it as a possible site for practice. Moreover, the quality of the educational experience may be improved by the presence of adequate clinical material in a locality.

There is a difference of opinion on the implications of a large number of vacant positions. Adams believes that competitive behavior would be furthered by a reduction in vacancies [104, p. 26]. The writer believes that vacancies help to create a seller's market and promote competition in the quality of educational programs [174, p. 206].

Competition for house staff by means of stipend is generally frowned upon. Payment of "excessive salaries" is held to render suspect the quality of a hospital's educational program. Both Adams [104, pp. 17–18] and the writer [174, p. 209] concluded that the quality and reputation of a teaching program appear to be a more important factor in recruiting young physicians than the amount of stipend offered. Other factors being equal, however, the stipend is important in many instances. It may be decisive for the outcome when the young physician's financial resources fall short of his family obligations.

It is believed that higher stipends during training might serve to lower the ultimate expectations of physicians for income. Higher stipends are also likely to discourage some hospitals in the quest for house staff and may lead to the partial substitution of paid-for services by physicians and technicians.

E. ESTIMATES OF SHORTAGE

What does a shortage of personnel mean to an economist? If price (income) is held below its equilibrium level, demand (the quantity people are willing to buy) will exceed supply (the quantity people offer for sale), and one observes a shortage in its most obvious form—vacancies. If actual price is above equilibrium price, then in a free market supply should exceed demand. If the excess is not observed, it may be presumed that supply is being limited through artificial means. Again, there is a shortage [Letter from Kenneth J. Arrow, February 2, 1962].

Evidence on income alone (or income in relation to the cost of entering an occupation) does not tell one how to combat a shortage. In the first of the above cases, the shortage is attributable to low income or is at least associated with it. In the second case the shortage is evidenced by high income.

Friedman-Kuznets Approach

Today's sophisticated analyses of professional income derive from Friedman and Kuznets, as do the applications to problems of manpower policy. They found that the average (arithmetic mean) annual income of physicians exceeded that of dentists by 32 percent [124, p. 105]. (In itself a difference in income between two professions does not establish a lack of adjustment between supply and demand, just as equal incomes would not be evidence of a close adjustment. It will be recalled that income in one occupation may be considerably higher than in another, in order to compensate for certain nonpecuniary disadvantages and for higher costs of training or to induce enough persons to enter the former occupation in order to meet a rising demand for services [124, p. 98].) Allowance for the higher costs of physician training (mostly income foregone) reduced the estimated equilibrium differential to 17 percent [124, p. 126]. Noting that greater variability of income among physicians probably made it the more attractive occupation and that such nonpecuniary advantages as prestige, opportunity to render service and make contacts, conditions of work, and so forth, also favored medicine [124, p. 130], Friedman and Kuznets concluded that the persistent income differential between the two related professions could only be explained if there were barriers to entry into medicine. Since they ruled out lack of persons with the requisite innate ability, the barriers could take the form of either limitations on the capacity of educational facilities or impediments to the granting of licenses by the states, or both [124, pp. 136–37]. Limitation of entry before admission to a professional school entails lower costs to society without any return than limitations at the stage of licensure.

On the basis of the inadequate data available Friedman and Kuznets calculated that there should be roughly three times as many physicians as dentists in order to eliminate the excessive income differential between the professions [124, p. 133]. At the time of their study the ratio of physicians to dentists was 2.1 [124, p. 29].

Friedman has elaborated on this analysis more recently. In medicine there is no significant way to effect direct control over fees or the annual income of physicians. Limitation of supply is the only practicable way to raise physicians' fees [11, p. 159]. The limitation is accomplished through control over the state licensure machinery, which is generally placed in the hands of the profession being licensed. The profession almost invariably seeks to employ the licensing machinery for the purpose of limiting entry [11, pp. 160–61] (and reducing the number of potential competitors).

Friedman has no doubt that the medical profession has effected a restriction of entry. Yet the restriction has served to raise average income above the equilibrium level by only 15–20 percent. The reason for the relatively small result, in his opinion, is the possibility and pervasiveness of economic substitution in the long run. He cites the growth of chiropractors, faith healers, and osteopaths [11, p. 159] (but makes no reference to the current tendency to upgrade the last).

Since the income differential between physicians and other professions has widened in the postwar period [42, pp. 204–5], some economists believe that the shortage of physicians persists or has become intensified [36a, p. 95]. This position may be based on the implicit assumption that the other variables that enter the Friedman-Kuznets analysis would not significantly alter the results derived from a comparison of the average income figures; or on the concept of a manpower shortage developed by Blank and Stigler, namely, that a shortage exists when the supply of workers increases less rapidly than the number demanded at wages or salaries received in the recent past, with the result that wages or salaries rise [110, p. 24].

In appraising the conclusions stated above, several questions may be asked.

1. How reliable are the income data? Nobody really knows [88, p. 26]. This is true despite the close agreement reported by most surveys of physician income [106, p. 222]. Friedman and Kuznets inquired into possible bias in response rate and in reporting of income. They concluded that response bias, while not large, probably involved underrepresentation of lower income physicians. Bias in reporting did not appear to be serious but probably made for an understatement of net income [124, pp. 445–46]. The two sources of bias tended to offset one another.

Representativeness of sample apart, it is clear that close agreement among surveys is compatible with both truthful reporting of income and with its systematic falsification. Perhaps data gathered for one purpose, such as a basis for setting fees, would yield a higher average income than data gathered for another purpose, such as taxation. Nevertheless, it is worth noting that data compiled from an audit of individual tax returns by the Internal Revenue Service Show that physicians underreport income to the same extent as other independent professions [119, p. 258]; the audit raised physicians' gross receipts by less than 2 percent and their net income by 8 percent. A major factor in the understatement of physicians' net income is the possibility of charging off as business expenses certain types of consumption expenditure [126, p. 85].

Comparison between aggregates of gross income based on surveys of physicians and of consumers shows the latter to be appreciably larger. After differences in definition were reconciled and an allowance was made for losses on collections, a difference of 10 percent remained [75a, p. 57]. It is not known whether, and by how much, consumers tend to exaggerate their expenditures for physician services.

The strongest views on the accuracy of physicians' income figures are expressed by Sanders, who believes that the published figures are too low [224, pp. 321–22]. He cites as evidence the existence of large numbers of vacancies in health departments with salary levels approaching and even exceeding the mean salary estimate employed by the U.S. Department of Commerce. Pointing to the advantages attached to such salaried positions, including shorter and more regular working hours and retirement benefits, and to the relatively low qualifications required of applicants, he concludes that the large numbers of vacancies reported would not exist if the data on physicians' income were correct. He neglects the fact that the vacant positions in public health often carry administrative duties, which many clinicians are not prepared or not willing to assume.

The Health Insurance Plan of New York has experienced difficulty in recruiting physicians for family practice at salaries that exceed the nation-wide average income and, therefore, the New York City average [174, p. 147]. It may be that some physicians are willing to pay a price for engaging in independent solo practice. This would be one of the nonpecuniary attractions of a particular way of life or the price of adhering to certain conventional beliefs of the medical profession.

If the income of physicians is actually higher than reported, the shortage of physicians is larger than calculated. If income is more accurately reported today than formerly [126, p. 84], owing to the increasing pervasiveness of the individual income tax and improvement in its collection and auditing machinery, then the rise in income over time has been overstated, and the change in the shortage position may be smaller than indicated.

2. Friedman and Kuznets themselves pointed to a possible source of error in their findings, namely, an understatement of the duration of training for specialty practice in medicine [124, p. 121]. They were writing at a time of rapid transition from preparation for a specialty via apprenticeship of practitioners to preparation via formal residency programs.

Friedman has recently suggested that his original analysis neglected the effect of the individual income tax [11, p. 220]. A progressive income tax collects more revenue from the occupation with the more variable and more widely fluctuating income. It also enhances the value of the nonpecuniary (hence untaxed) advantages of an occupation. In the case of physicians the two factors operate in opposite directions.

3. The measure of the cost of postponed income is heavily affected by the rate of discount chosen. Is it not possible that the medical student's time preference is higher than the prevailing market rate of interest, on the ground that his postponement of income is accompanied by personal and family decisions that have enduring consequences and are not reversible? The rate of return on private investment in education is substantially higher than the 4 percent figure employed by Friedman and Kuznets [136a, pp. 118–19]. (See Chapter VII, Section B.)

4. Is the mean annual income of a profession a more appropriate measure of remuneration than income per hour? On the average, practicing physicians work long hours—perhaps 60 hours a week. This is, of course, a longer work week than that of factory workers or plumbers. Inclusive of time spent at conferences and professional reading, how does it compare with the work week in other self-employed professions?

5. What sets the level of equilibrium income for the medical profession? Is it derived through comparisons with incomes and costs of other comparable professions after (downward) allowance is made for the undeniable attractions of medicine as an occupation; or should one recognize with Adam Smith that the reward of physicians must be such "as may give them that rank in society which so important a trust requires" [40, p. 105]? The importance consumers attach to physicians' services contributes to the inelasticity of demand [124, p. 139]. Does this factor have

implications for the level of income of physicians, as well as for its dispersion [43b, p. 199]?

6. How relevant is the actuarial test (comparison of expected average incomes) for an occupation that can exercise some control over its income through the ability to prescribe the number of services rendered? A physician who is hard-pressed financially is in a position to prescribe additional visits and procedures [140, p. 8].

It does not follow, of course, that society has no practical means for eliminating a calculated shortage of physicians. Rather, one must proceed with caution in taking corrective measures. Moreover, it might be sensible to set the goal short of competitive equilibrium.

Conclusions Reached by Other Economists

Other economists have dealt with the problem of physician shortage, either purposefully and systematically or incidentally to other concerns. Among the former Hansen's recent work warrants recognition.

Drawing initially on Friedman and Kuznets, Hansen estimates the rates of return to be expected from investment in alternative types of professional training, especially medicine and dentistry. He takes into consideration both the cost and return dimensions of professional career choices [126, p. 75] and solves for that internal rate of return that equates the present value of the expected earnings stream to the present value of the expected outlay or cost stream. He then compares the rates of return in medicine and in dentistry with some standard, or equilibrium, level [126, p. 82]—say, the rate earned by all male college graduates [126, p. 85]. A deviation of 5 percent (one twentieth) or more from the equilibrium rate is designated a shortage if positive, and a surplus if negative.

In 1939 the internal rates of return for physicians and for dentists fell short of the equilibrium rate, indicating a surplus for each. By 1949 the situation was reversed, with shortages indicated for both. The major reason was the decline in the equilibrium rate of return. Between 1949 and 1956 the rates of return for both physicians and dentists fell, owing largely to the rise in costs of training. Although there was still a sizable shortage of physicians, the shortage of dentists was slight [126, p. 86]. (The 1956 rates of return for male college graduates, physicians, and dentists were, respectively, 11.6, 12.8, and 12.0 percent.)

Hansen concludes that the financial rewards of medicine have declined, so that the importance attached to restrictions on entry (traceable to Friedman and Kuznets) may have been misplaced [126, p. 89]. He cites the apparent decline in the number and quality of medical school applicants in support of his conclusion [126, p. 75] but offers no evidence. Much depends on the base line selected, for a considerable decline in the number of applicants set in with the departure of World War II veterans from the schools in the early 1950s. However, by and large, the aptitudes of those currently admitted to medical school are equal or superior to those admitted in the past [133, p. 123].

Other economists have pointed to certain facts as obviously indicative of a shortage of physicians.

1. Today one of two applicants to medical school is denied admission. There is no reason to believe that all or most of the rejected applicants are unqualified to pursue a medical career. In fact, Friedman and Kuznets showed that the proportion accepted was no lower among those applying for admission to medical school a second or third time, after prior rejection, than among those applying the first time [124, p. 15]. To some economists the persistence of a large number of rejected, but qualified, applicants constitutes clear proof of a shortage [36a, p. 104].

If it is assumed that most applicants who are rejected would succeed in passing the medical school course, a possible rebuttal to the above argument is to emphasize the expensiveness of medical education. If society were aware of the true costs, would it be willing to train everybody for medicine who wanted such training [149, p. 256]? Moreover, since tuition fees do not cover the cost to the school, should the returns from the public investment accrue to individual physicians or be distributed otherwise in a socially advantageous way [124, pp. vi–vii]? Should not medical students be expected to pay a much larger share of the cost, out of borrowed funds, if necessary [87, p.

145]? If so, might not unrestricted entry under the changed conditions yield smaller numbers of students than at present? The average quality of students would probably decline [55, p. 956].

2. The reported ratio of physicians per 100,000 population has fluctuated around 133 for a long time, while national income (or gross national product) and expenditures for health and medical care have increased substantially. Is a constant personnel ratio compatible?

On the one hand, the present ratio is lower than the ratio of 150–160 that obtained sixty years ago, when the medical diploma mills were prominent. Today's physician is better qualified, however, and the numbers graduated from American medical schools have continued to increase in the postwar period.

On the other hand, this country's physician-to-population ratio is higher than that in most countries. Only Israel and Russia exceed the United States ratio, at 238 and 172, respectively [47, p. 34].

To determine the implications of trends in the physician-to-population ratio, it is necessary to compare trends in the productivity of physicians and in the demand for their services. This task has not yet been performed satisfactorily.

The improvement in productivity, as calculated from certain economic time series (see Chapter VII, Section A), has furnished a basis for denying a shortage of physicians and for raising the possibility of a potential surplus [117, p. 14]. The latter could ensue if the demand for physician services remained constant and the proportion of practicing to total physicians did not change.

In fact the demand for physician services has increased, and consumers use more services per capita. In addition, more physicians spend more time on activities other than patient care.

3. Vacancies in hospital house staffs and the large number of foreign physicians serving as interns and residents in this country are frequently adduced as proof of a shortage of physicians [4, p. 161; 42, p. 123]. An alternative criterion, derived from Blank and Stigler and pointing to the same conclusion, was employed in an economic analysis of the intern market, namely, that in recent years salaries have risen faster for interns than for other occupations [104, pp. 13–15].

Neither fact would, however, be pertinent evidence concerning a shortage of physicians, if members of hospital house staffs were receiving training exclusively; in that case the sole contribution of a training program would be to help improve the quality of care or to raise the prestige of an institution. Owing to the low stipends paid to house staff, it is not surprising that hospitals always want more of them. (Of 202 hospital intern programs that lapsed, only 17 withdrew voluntarily.) Moreover, it is the policy of the responsible authorities in graduate medical education to pass only on the educational potential of a program and not to seek to equalize the total numbers of training positions and applicants in the country.

In fact a portion of the services performed by house staff is essential for patient care, in the sense that in their absence other physicians and auxiliary personnel would be required to perform them. However, since the services of house staff are underpaid (hence economically undervalued), the criterion of vacancies would overstate the size of the potential replacement problem. The real questions are whether practicing physicians, especially young ones, have sufficient slack time to assume the service assignment; and, if so, whether their reputations would suffer if they accepted remuneration.

Techniques Employed in Public Health and Medical Care

Authorities in public health and medical care estimate the magnitude of the physician shortage by subtracting the projected number of available physicians from the number required. Estimating the former is simple, for few physicians leave the profession for other work and the entry route is strictly controlled by licensure [139, pp. 222–24]. Requirements are estimated by adopting as a standard one or another physician-to-population ratio.

The several variants of this approach to estimating physician requirements fall into two groups: (a) need, a standard set by professional judgment and (b) present utilization, a datum derived from the vast body of available statistics on health and medical manpower.

The classic treatment of need as a standard for calculating

manpower requirements is by Lee and Jones in the monograph they wrote for the Committee on the Cost of Medical Care. Drawing on the best current information on the expectancy (incidence or prevalence) of diseases and injuries, they proceeded to estimate the number of physician hours required to prevent, diagnose, and treat each major disease and injury category according to the prevailing consensus of leading members of the health professions. Requirements for physician hours were converted into requirements for physicians on the basis that the average physician devotes 2,000 hours a year to caring for patients. It was found that a population of 100,000 requires 135 physicians for the individual care of patients [134, p. 115].

The Lee-Jones study is now thirty-five years old and has not been repeated. Some economists sympathize with this approach, that of substituting professional judgment for consumer choice as the guide for policy in a field in which the market works imperfectly [161, pp. 116, 128].

Others, including the writer, hold a more critical view of the standard of need. This approach would be applicable if we had the technical knowledge for translating figures on the expectancy of diseases and injuries into requirements for services; if we could agree on the number of services—or even hours of service—rendered per physician per year; if we accepted health as an absolute goal of society and physicians' services as a fixed factor in promoting this goal; and if we were willing and able as individuals, communities, or as a nation, to underwrite financially uniform standards of adequate (or minimum) medical services throughout the country, without regard to other objects of expenditure, necessary or desired [130, pp. 634, 644]. None of these provisos seems to obtain today.

It is of historical interest that the final estimates of Lee and Jones were mistaken in terms of their own data. For the individual care of patients the calculated need was for 165,400 physicians. This figure was compared with 152,500 [134, pp. 114–15], the number listed in the directory of the American Medical Association in 1929. The computed deficit of 12,900 physicians represents a serious understatement, for the supply figure includes inactive as well as retired physicians; and the need figure fails to allow for additional requirements for tuberculosis and mental sanitoriums, public health, medical education, and medical research. One may surmise that a small deficit was perhaps more congenial to the temper of the 1930s than a large one.

Methods that begin with an existing physician-to-population ratio have some advantages over the criterion of need, but they are also vulnerable to additional criticisms. Determining requirements for physicians by applying to the nation the ratio of physicians to population experienced by the aggregate of the top twelve states avoids the objection that we do not know how to proceed from morbidity data to physician requirements, but it is clearly subject to the other criticisms stated above. Moreover, this method of calculating requirements is suspect insofar as it is almost bound to yield a shortage [117, p. 8].

Determining requirements by setting the standard at some point in an array of physician-to-population ratios (such as 50 states or 120 trading areas) becomes decreasingly vulnerable to these criticisms with a reduction in the standard; and conversely. But under this method of calculating requirements, success achieved in overcoming an estimated shortage today might conceivably serve to increase the shortage calculated tomorrow. Moreover, the method is mechanical and does not deal with the changes that occur in the real world [126, p. 7]. It cannot be said to yield a valid criterion in the absence of a field test, such as the following: does the ratio selected as the standard derive from a geographic area that may be said to be reasonably representative, in the sense that it provides acceptable levels of care without an extra large contingent of physicians in medical education and research?

Another application of the physician-to-population ratio for determining future requirements assumes that the number of physicians should be large enough to maintain the national ratio in a selected base year, to make up well-defined deficiencies, and to meet important requirements likely to develop in the foreseeable future [29, Vol. 2, pp. 184–85]. This method, which was originally employed in World War II, is useful for mobilization planning. For the purpose of long-range planning in a civilian economy the method has been criticized on several grounds: no evidence is submitted that the base year selected was optimal in any sense; the results of the calculations tend to be taken too literally, so that a big expansion program is based on a small estimate of shortage; a projected requirement that allows only for an increase in population is conservative, so that a shortage may ensue even if the proposed program is fully implemented [126, p. 78].

Eclectic Approaches

Two attempts have been made to study the problem of physician shortage through the application of more eclectic approaches drawing on knowledge of both economics and medical care. Neither one developed numerical answers but sought to determine the directions that manpower policy might properly pursue.

In 1950 the writer concluded that the market cannot test the adequacy of the number of physicians, if need is accepted as the basis for determining requirements for medical care. However, professional medical criteria alone will not suffice, for economic costs, in the sense of alternatives foregone, must be taken into account. At the time, it was proposed that the most practical method for ascertaining a standard of need is to study the utilization experience of known populations who receive comprehensive medical services by paying moderate insurance premiums. It was noted that any standard of need must be financially underwritten, in order to avoid idleness of the resources provided in accordance with the standard. From a technical standpoint, it was urged that the emphasis be not on projecting future requirements but on developing methods, techniques, and data that will enable one to estimate requirements currently, under alternative policy assumptions [130, pp. 644–45].

The National Manpower Council approached the problem broadly, with major concern for the quality of care. After analyzing the quantitative estimates of physician requirements calculated by public health authorities and finding them wanting, it proceeded to list and discuss the factors pointing toward an increased demand for physicians' services. The conclusion was that specific shortages were evident in certain specialties, such as psychiatry, public health, and pathology. Moreover, the Council concluded that, regardless of actuarial calculations, physicians' incomes were obviously high enough to enable them to exercise some discretion in choosing the time and the place of practice. The view was expressed that an increase in the number of new recruits to the profession would facilitate desired changes at the margin. In addition, the Council proposed improving the utilization of the existing number of physicians and noted the obstacle to efficient utilization posed by the requirement of specialty boards that young physicians limit their practice to a single field [139, pp. 239–40].

The Council stressed the distinction between long-run, or structural, shortages and transitional shortages resulting from a sudden expansion of demand. Both their consequences and remedies differ [139, p. 155].

Geographic Distribution

Data showing higher physician-to-population ratios in urban areas than in rural areas and in high income areas than in low income areas are commonplace [107, pp. 80–81; 155, Chapter 1, p. 17]. These findings have been challenged on two grounds: the physician-to-population ratio is a meaningless measure of supply [197, pp. 3–5]; there are few people in this country (one sixth of 1 percent) who are not within 25 miles of a practicing physician [118, p. 3].

The fact remains, however, that economic factors do influence a physician's choice of a specific community in which to settle [120, p. 214]. As a result, the population of low income areas have less access to physicians. The work load of their physicians is greater and average time per patient visit is shorter [141, p. 12]. Persons of low or moderate income in these areas have the further disadvantage of not being able to travel for care elsewhere [92, p. 680].

It is expected that an increase in the total number of physicians would serve to attract part of the increment to areas with low physician to population ratios. However, the well-to-do areas would fare even better [141, p. 12]. One solution is to increase the number of doctors with rural backgrounds and orientations [139, p. 238]. Another is to underwrite a national minimum by financing it [130, p. 645]. Still another is to allow time to realize the long-run tendency for regional differences in income to diminish [141, p. 12]. There is apparently little to gain from increased mobility on a voluntary basis, for the present distribution of physicians reflects fairly free migration [87, p. 152].

Present Consensus

As a practical matter, there now exists a broad consensus on policy in this country, shared by the American Medical Association, that with the projected increase in population the number of physicians must increase [42, pp. 124–25]. For this to occur ten to thirty four-year medical schools are to be established. To the writer, the bases on which the consensus was reached are not evident.

The proposition that more medical graduates means more medical schools, almost in strict proportion, is seldom questioned. Millett is perhaps the outstanding exception in asking whether we might not abandon the traditional emphasis on small classes in medical school, associated with individual instruction, and make efforts to improve the productivity of medical education [138, pp. 186–88]. It is a fact, perhaps little known, that a significant fraction of the postwar expansion in total output by American medical schools has occurred in existing medical schools. A study of how this was accomplished—the increases in staff and facilities that were prerequisite—would be useful.

V. SUPPLY OF HOSPITAL SERVICES

However measured—whether in terms of capital investment, operating expenditures, the number of employees, the seriousness of the illnesses cared for, the effect on the pattern of medical care organization, or the contribution to medical education and medical research—the hospital is the major facility in the health and medical care industry. It is also the object of a great deal of public attention and professional study.

A. THE HOSPITAL'S ROLE

The modern hospital is not long removed from its antecedents—the pest house, almshouse, and shelter for the sick poor. Only the advent of antiseptic surgery and asepsis in the last quarter of the nineteenth century eliminated the need to destroy hospital pavilions infected with "hospitalitis." Hospitals then became fit to care for the middle classes and the well-to-do as inpatients (occupants of beds), if not as outpatients. Continued technological advances in medicine, along with the rise in the national income and the subsequent growth of insurance for hospital care, expanded the hospital's part in serving the entire population. In the past fifty years the formal education of the physician has extended in this country to more than 1,000 hospitals outside the immediate purview of the medical school, and in the period since World War II the expansion of medical research has increased the volume of clinical research performed in hospitals.

The several programs of the hospital have evolved at uneven rates, a situation that has led to a divergence of opinion regarding the institution's true objectives and essential missions. In the *Encyclopedia Britannica* Rufus Rorem has defined the hospital as follows: "It is a place where sick and injured persons

receive medical care of such nature that some patients are required to utilize a bed during part or all of their stay." Other
definitions list among the hospital's functions the care of patients, medical education, and research [171, p. 11]. Brown has
presented a general definition that attempts to capture the social
and economic nature of the institution: "A hospital is the community's centralized facilities for medical care. It represents a
cooperative effort whereby the total community has pooled its
resources in order to provide the sorts of specialized equipment
and highly trained personnel that no patient or doctor could provide individually, and which no patient could afford to use and
maintain by himself" [113, p. 24]. Emphasis is sometimes put
on the hospital's role as the community health center that serves
all segments of the population and promotes the health of the individual patient.

There are approximately 7,000 hospitals in this country,
with 1.7 million beds. Since there is no simple way to measure
the volume of other types of equipment in the hospital, the bed
is treated in a manner analogous to the division slice in the
military, standing for both a part of the nursing unit (accommo-
dating patients) and a proportionate share of all the other facilities [176, p. 212]. The correlation between the number of beds and
facilities such as the X-ray department is probably closer than
that between the number of beds and some of the other facilities,
such as the outpatient department.

The hospitals in this country embody an investment of $19.1
billion, spend $9.4 billion annually, and employ 1.7 million per-
sons [105, p. 414]. Associated with them are more than 300,000
non-employees, including physicians, private duty nurses, trustees, and volunteers [131, pp. 71-72].

Of primary interest to the public are the 5,700 short-term
hospitals. With 44 percent of all beds, they admit 94 percent of
the 25.5 million inpatients, provide almost all of the outpatient
and emergency services rendered by hospitals, and account for
67 percent of the capital investment in hospitals and 73 percent
of the annual expenditures. Among short-term hospitals the general hospital is predominant.

Most general hospitals are concerned with the treatment of

short-term patients with acute illness [42, p. 64]. The care of long-term patients with chronic diseases, of ambulatory patients, or of patients at home ranks secondary among their priorities.

Notwithstanding, general hospitals are important. Here all major surgery is performed and much minor surgery. Most births occur within their walls. Here also takes place much of medical diagnosis, especially of inpatients; considerable medical treatment that requires either daily attendance by a physician or regular nursing care; and an increasing proportion of all emergency services rendered by physicians. Here, too, the unexpected, very large medical bill is incurred.

B. SHAPE AND LEVEL OF SUPPLY CURVES

Strictly speaking the concept of a supply function (or curve) applies only to a competitive industry. In practice the tool may be useful even when considerable departures from the rigorous criteria of pure competition occur [43a, p. 216].

The supply curve of an industry is the horizontal sum of the marginal cost curves of the individual firms. This is true in the long run, as well as in the short run. The only difference due to length of run—a difference that makes for serious complications in analysis—is that in the long run the number of firms must also be determined [43b, p. 172].

Underlying any supply curve are certain givens, as previously noted (Chapter IV, Section A). When any of these conditions change, the curve is said to have shifted.

This section deals with three topics:

1. The shapes of the cost curves of the individual hospital and of the industry in the short run, when the size of each hospital and the number of hospitals are fixed and only certain inputs may be varied.

2. The shapes of the cost curves of the individual hospital and of the industry in the long run, when both the size of hospital and the number of hospitals may vary.

3. The factors responsible for the rising trend in hospital cost (the upward shift in the hospital's cost curves).

Short Run

Feldstein performed an intensive study of the departmental costs of one hospital in relation to variations in its patient load. He found that the functional form of the relationships between total cost and output (patient days, mostly) could best be represented by means of linear regression analysis [121, p. 14]; he searched for other (curvilinear) forms of relationship but could not find them [121, p. 56]. Linearity of total cost implies that marginal cost is constant over the observed range of output. (Expressed mathematically, marginal cost is the first derivative of total cost.)

In economic theory the short-run marginal cost curve is conceived to be upward sloping, owing to the onset of diminishing returns when one or more factors of production are fixed while others vary. However, most statistical studies of cost curves in industry yield a short-run marginal cost curve that is horizontal (infinitely elastic) over the usual range of output. One possible explanation lies in unused capacity [11, p. 138]. Feldstein considered this explanation and dismissed it on the ground that the rate of occupancy in the hospital he studied was high—90 percent [121, p. 62].

The other possibility, suggested by Stigler, is that a horizontal marginal cost curve for a firm is the necessary outcome of its quest for flexibility. If a firm's rate of output were foreseeable and fixed, the goal would be to minimize the cost of the projected volume of output. Since a firm's rate of output varies, owing to fluctuations in demand, its objective is to employ techniques that are tolerably efficient (and do not yield large differences in cost) over a probable range of outputs. Flexibility is not a free good, for the cost of producing any stated rate of output is higher in a flexible plant than it would be in a plant designed precisely for that output [43b, p. 118].

If the supply curve of the individual hospital is horizontal, the supply curve of the industry is also horizontal [43b, pp. 166–67]. (The exceptions to this proposition are not important.)

Feldstein conducted separate studies of 16 component accounts (or departments) in the hospital. For some accounts, such as supply expense, food, drugs, and unskilled labor, he found costs to be responsive to variations in the number of patient days. Accounts in which costs do not respond to variations in patient days include plant, equipment, and several categories of skilled and specialized personnel. The costs of registered nurses, laboratory and X-ray technicians, and administrative personnel do not vary in the short run. At prevailing salaries the hospital is not able to hire registered nurses when they are needed, so it hires them when they are available. Registered nurses are graduated in September; as many as are willing are then recruited in anticipation of the attrition that will take place throughout the forthcoming year. In the case of technicians costs of training are entailed, and the hospital prefers to retain those it has hired [121, pp. 52–53].

Some degree of variation in staffing with registered nurses is introduced through the employment of per diem nurses. More informally, patients and their physicians may be induced to hire private duty nurses when the demand for nursing care is high. The numbers involved can be large, and in some hospitals the number of private duty nurses exceeds the number of registered nurses on general duty [174, p. 240].

For the hospital in its entirety Feldstein found that marginal cost is one quarter (21 to 27 percent) of average cost per patient day [121, p. 49]. Thus, the marginal cost of an additional patient day in an existing hospital is relatively small. It is a mathematical truth that as long as marginal cost is less than average cost, the latter must be declining. This is, in turn, consistent with Feldstein's finding that the long-run average cost curve for hospitals is also declining [121, p. 2].

Long Run

For his study of the long-run (or complete) adaptation of the hospital to variations in patient load Feldstein used data from 60 hospitals. He found the marginal cost curve to be constant, that is, there was no difference in patient day cost between small hospitals and large ones. Since large hospitals offer the wider range of services, the long-run marginal cost curve may be said to display a downward slope.

In this case, too, marginal cost is less than average cost,

as indicated by the presence of a positive constant term in the equation for total cost. It follows that the long-run average cost curve must be falling. This means that for the size of hospitals included in the sample—48 to 453 beds—economies of scale exist throughout the entire range [121, pp. 63–64].

Feldstein's results are not consistent with those of other studies. In the 1930s the Hospital Survey for New York found a curvilinear relationship between the average patient day cost and the size of hospital [129, p. 343]. More recent data for the New York area display a similar U-shaped pattern [142, p. 31]. The findings of the Commission on Financing Hospital Care, which show a high correlation between the range of services and the patient day cost, are similar [127, pp. 107, 112].

A U-shaped cost curve for the long run is plausible. At a sufficiently small output, efficiency increases with size, owing chiefly to the specialization of labor and equipment. At sufficiently larger outputs, efficiency declines with size because of increasing complexities of management [43b, p. 140]. In hospitals two additional factors reinforce this outcome. At the lower end of the size scale average patient day cost is increased by a low rate of occupancy. (This effect is commonly ascribed to the tendency for patient day census to follow a random process, described by the Poisson distribution. In this statistical distribution the standard deviation is equal to the square root of the arithmetic mean [157, p. 76].) As the size of the hospital increases, cost tends to be raised by the provision of a wider range of services and sometimes also by expanded teaching programs.

The discrepancy between Feldstein's and other findings may be due in part to differences in the characteristics of the hospitals studied, with special reference to the range of services and the scope of the teaching program. In addition, his substitution of patient days for bed capacity as the independent variable removes the influence of size on the rate of occupancy, especially in small hospitals. Finally, given the existence of specialized factors of production with diverse talent, including hospital administrators, medical staffs, and boards of trustees, there may be a range of optimum sizes, rather than a single optimum size [11, p. 142]. Possibly the bottom of the U-shaped curve is flat.

A U-shaped average cost curve is associated with an upward sloping marginal cost curve that intersects its lowest point. Where average cost is constant, marginal cost is also constant.

An econometric study of the behavior of hospital cost in the long run, with special reference to the effects of size and occupancy, is under way at the University of Michigan [148].

The long-run supply curve of the industry will have a shape and position determined by two factors: the shape of the marginal cost curves of individual hospitals; and the conditions of entry (and departure) for new (existing) hospitals. If the individual hospitals have highly elastic supply (marginal cost) curves, the industry's supply curve will be virtually horizontal, even in the absence of entry by new firms. If the individual marginal cost curves rise rapidly, the industry's supply curve can still be highly elastic if there are many potential new hospitals [43b, p. 173].

The number of existing hospitals depends on the conditions governing entry and departure, or closure. In the business sector profits attract and losses repel. In the hospital field a decisive factor is the type of ownership. This is of sufficient importance to warrant separate discussion (in the next section).

Rise in Hospital Cost

The short-run supply curve holds these things constant: the size of the facility; techniques of production; and the prices of factors of production. For the long-run supply curve the first item is allowed to vary, but the other two continue to be fixed [11, pp. 75–76]. When techniques of production or the prices of factors change, the cost curve is said to have shifted.

Damrau lists three major explanations of hospital cost increases: (a) the closing of the gap in wages and working conditions between hospitals and other industries; (b) the increasing complexity and costliness of hospital care, due to medical advances; and (c) the hospitals' lag in productivity gains behind the economy at large [116, pp. 202–3]. From a technical (economic) standpoint explanations (*a*) and (*c*) fall in the same category, a change in the prices of factors of production. The difference between them is that explanation (*a*) posits a one time adjustment (or discontinuous adjustments) while explanation (*c*) is consistent with continuing shifts in the curve.

The writer inquired into hospital cost increases in one large city (New York City). The closing-the-gap explanation seemed plausible immediately after World War II [125, p. 60] but is not consistent with developments throughout most of the period 1948–1957. At the close of this period hospital wages were still low.

Advances in medical knowledge or technique often lead to higher cost, as more can be, and is, done for the patient [32, pp. 55, 105]. Criteria of what constitutes good medical care are constantly reappraised and revised, usually upward. For most illnesses higher cost is implied by an increase in the number of procedures per patient stay and per patient day.

A prominent manifestation of medical progress in the postwar period is the reduction that occurred in the average duration of patient stay. Some advances, such as early ambulation after surgery or childbirth, entail no additional expenditures and progress is costless. Associated with a reduced stay, however, is the concentration of certain diagnostic and major therapeutic services over a shorter interval, thereby raising the average level of activity in the hospital.

Average duration of stay ceased to decline in the middle 1950s and has actually increased in some instances, while hospital cost continued to rise. The cessation of the downward trend in stay reflects in part the achievement of a relatively low death rate in the hospital for most diagnostic groups and the aging of the hospital population. Aged patients stay longer in the general hospital than other patients, but contrary to expectations appear to use more services per patient day [122, pp. 59, 63].

When expressed quantitatively, the medical progress explanation frequently takes the form of a comparison in the respective rates of increase of the several components of hospital cost, such as ancillary services and the so-called "hotel" services. The former show much higher rates of increase than the latter [132, pp. 233–34].

For studying the factors that underlie the upward shift in the hospital cost curve, it seems more appropriate to compare the respective contributions of the several major departmental groupings of the hospital to the total increase in its patient day cost. The writer found that the increase in special professional services (laboratory, radiology, and the surgical and maternity suites) was the same as in nursing, each contributing less than one fourth of the dollar increase in patient day cost. Other general professional services, including drugs, medical records, social work, and house staff, contributed 15 percent of the total increase; this is not appreciably more than was contributed by housekeeping, laundry, and plant maintenance. The dollar increase in expenditures for administration, fringe benefits, insurance, and so forth, was only slightly less than the increase in special hospital services, the hospital's diagnostic and treatment facilities *par excellence*.

The third explanation, that of a lag in productivity gains behind the rest of the economy, is accepted as an important factor by most economists who have thought about, or dealt with, hospital cost [51, p. 144; 160, p. 189; 202, p. 7]. That hospitals lag in productivity gains is supported by one of the few studies of productivity (defined as output per unit of labor input) that compares trends in hospitals and in other service fields. Among eight agencies or major components of agencies in the federal government only one—the Veterans Administration hospitals—failed to register an increase in productivity [137, pp. 351–52].

This explanation has serious implications. In general, wages tend to move with productivity gains in the economy at large. Wage rates for the same occupation are more or less competitive among industries. The wages paid by an industry are not limited by the absence of productivity gains in that industry. Where possibilities for achieving gains in productivity are limited, as in hospitals, higher wages signify higher cost. Paradoxically, "any improvement in the productivity of labor in general will adversely affect hospital costs [112, p. 37]."

The writer also considered other explanations. Several factors, including the rising cost of nursing education, house staff education, and the employment of full-time chiefs of clinical service, jointly account for approximately 10 percent of the increase in patient day cost in the 1950s [132, pp. 239–41].

It should be noted that a hospital's cost data are for care furnished *by* the hospital, not *in* the hospital. Exclusion of the expenditures for private duty nurses has been noted. Certain other changes have occurred, which suggest the possibility that the upward shift in the cost curve may be understated. A good example of this phenomenon is the transfer of the anesthesia function from the nurse (a hospital employee) to the physician anesthesiologist (an independent practitioner who presents the patient with a separate bill).

C. OWNERSHIP: DETERMINANT OF SIZE AND NUMBER OF HOSPITALS

It has been noted that proprietary (for profit) hospitals provide a small fraction of hospital services in the United States and are concentrated in a few metropolitan areas. Government hospitals play a larger part numerically, but their total volume of services is the sum of services furnished to several special groups, rather than to a representative cross section of a community's population. In most areas it is the voluntary (nonprofit) hospital that serves the population at large, with the hospital owned by the state medical school affording the major exception.

Proprietary Hospitals

There is a widely held conviction in this country, especially among persons in the health field, that the proprietary form of hospital ownership is not socially desirable [161, p. 18]. The reasons for disapproval vary. To begin with, there is the strong feeling that nobody should make a profit from sickness [55, p. 950]. The physician's bill is regarded as a professional fee and not as business income. It is believed that a proprietary institution tends to skimp on services or supplies, particularly those of a scientific character about which the patient lacks knowledge and judgment. The absence of teaching programs for interns and residents, as well as for medical students, is seen as evidence of poor quality of care. Moreover, many proprietary hospitals do not qualify for accreditation by the Joint Commission on Accreditation of Hospitals, whose standards are intended to offer a minimum assurance of patients' safety.

One reason for lack of accreditation is small size; hospitals under 25 beds are not eligible. Most proprietary hospitals are small, a fact that usually implies a limited range of services and a low rate of occupancy. The latter means a waste of capital investment and an inefficient (high cost) operation. A hospital with a narrow range of services poses the danger that services of greater complexity will be attempted than lie within the capability of the institution and its staff.

Proprietary hospitals are sometimes criticized for "skimming off the cream," that is, caring for patients with simple diagnoses and uncomplicated courses of treatment and leaving to other hospitals the care of patients with the more complicated illnesses that are more difficult and more costly [146, p. 229]. Their physician-owners are believed to be in a position to reduce the patients' hospital charges below cost and to offset them, if necessary, with a higher medical bill.

Most proprietary hospitals care only for semi-private, acutely ill patients, many of whom are covered by voluntary health insurance. They do not serve inpatients with long-term illness or patients who lack financial means. Nor do they serve ambulatory patients in organized outpatient departments or in emergency departments.

In behalf of the proprietary form of organization it can be argued that such hospitals usually meet a public need for facilities—the ultimate criterion for judging the social usefulness of any economic activity. Moreover, most proprietary hospitals are owned by physicians. How is the hospital's role to be distinguished from that of its physician-owners? The advocates of proprietary hospitals note that physicians on their staffs are professional persons who are legally licensed by the state. Indeed, the same physicians frequently practice both in proprietary hospitals and in voluntary or government hospitals. Is there any evidence that a given physician varies his standards of performance between institutions?

Proprietary hospitals have demonstrated an ability to respond to changing community needs by moving quickly to expand facilities or to relocate in response to population shifts. Some proprietary hospitals meet community needs other than that for the care of acute ill inpatients by providing limited emergency departments, and a few admit patients with tuberculosis and care for them at public expense. When voluntary hospitals deny staff appointments to certain groups of physicians with demonstrated qualifications, proprietary hospitals may allow them to admit patients [186, p. 210].

Given the strong feeling that exists against proprietary hospitals, it is possible that a cumulative self-selection process ultimately validates the criticisms. (This point was made by Kenneth Arrow.) It has also been suggested that exclusive reliance on revenues from patients is likely to result in curtailing the range and the quality of the services rendered [144, p. 9].

Where proprietary hospitals exist, they are tolerated, either on the ground of the public's current need for the facilities or for lack of a legal basis for eliminating them. They receive close supervision, however, sometimes under special statutes and regulations. The regulatory process is likely to be detailed and strict, producing irritation on the part of the regulated and a sense of futility among the regulators [172, p. 48].

Voluntary Hospitals

Although the voluntary (nonprofit) form of organization is not unique to the hospital field, it is uncommon in the American economy. Among the factors responsible for this form of hospital organization are the close link between medical service and medical education, the concern that various population groups have had to insure staff appointments for their physicians, and the relatively large masses of capital involved.

In contrast to the proprietary hospital are the advantages attributed to the voluntary hospital. Typically, the latter serves all income groups in a community, not only those who can pay.

As such, it possesses built-in flexibility against fluctuations in the population's income over the business cycle. It often provides such facilities as emergency departments, and sometimes it provides organized care in the home. The board of trustees of leading citizens represents the community and has ultimate responsibility for insuring the provision of care of adequate quality. The organized medical staff can be a potent instrument of supervision and control over the activities of its members, and its purview may extend outside the hospital's walls. The trustees control this instrument in behalf of the community through their authority to appoint, promote, and fire (by failing to renew an appointment), and can enforce upon physicians close adherence to the medical staff's standards. Where the community also participates in financing, more and better services can be provided, thereby helping to offset any tendency by the market to undervalue the benefits yielded by a hospital.

The truth is, of course, that not every voluntary hospital admits patients from all income classes, is managed by a strong and responsible board of trustees, and receives financial support from its community. Nor does every voluntary hospital train interns and residents. Nevertheless, a hospital with access to income from sources other than patients may possess superior facilities and more ample working capital, and therefore be less likely to skimp on services. Today medical education costs money [132, p. 239], and it is still conducted for the most part with medically indigent patients whose care the hospital may be required to subsidize. Finally, if the hospital is ever to serve as the community health center, it must care for bed patients and ambulatory patients from all income classes.

A possible defect of the voluntary form of organization is that the ordinary economic incentives to efficiency are lacking. Indeed, their very desirability has been questioned. It is asserted that nothing is too costly when human life is at stake [143, p. 10]. Furthermore, since nobody derives dividends from a nonprofit hospital, it is postulated that cost of production must be lower than in a similar institution conducted as a business [109]; in other words, the potential contribution of entrepreneurship is neglected. The possibility that inefficiency of operation may intrude is further excluded on the ground that trustees of voluntary hospitals are distinguished men of affairs who are devoted to the institution's interests [109]. Finally, with hospital administrators becoming better trained academically and more experienced, the danger of inefficient operation is said to have diminished [127, p. 50]. Thus, major reliance is placed on professional knowledge and personal integrity, and little need is seen for the external pressures and rewards that are applied in the business sector of the economy.

Notwithstanding, the writer believes that incentives to efficiency are not only desirable but needed. Although many voluntary hospitals apply management techniques, including budgets, the traditional division of authority and responsibility among the chief elements of management—trustees, physicians, and administration—sometimes hinders the development of a consistent set of goals and may interfere with singleness of purpose in moving toward their attainment. (See also Chapter V, Section D.)

Government Hospitals

To say that a service, such as hospital care, properly falls within the scope of government expenditures is not the same as to say that government will produce that service. It is frequently practicable for government to purchase it from private industry [2, p. 22; 16, p. 113; 23, p. 15]. What are, then, the criteria for determining whether government will produce a service it pays for or purchase it?

Unlike the administration of courts, the administration of hospitals is a type of activity that can appropriately be entrusted to private operation. Most economists would agree, therefore, that the decisive test for choosing between business and government ownership and operation (not financing) is comparative efficiency [2, p. 22]. The answer is qualified if accompanying costs of administration or regulation are substantial [34, pp. 361–62]. The efficiency test is irrelevant when private industry will not produce the service, as in the case of public health [56. p. 107].

The fact that government hospitals care for special groups in the population has served to link the production and the financing of services and to minimize their purchase. Thus, the Veterans Administration buys only small amounts of care from other institutions, and for many years the military services were reluctant to buy care for the dependents of military personnel. Local governments have traditionally paid for some care rendered in voluntary hospitals, but rates per patient day were low and criteria for certifying patients as public charges were strict. Even today many cities apply one set of criteria of eligibility (liberal) in their own hospitals and another (stringent) in voluntary hospitals. Uniform application of criteria is increasingly likely to obtain, however, and the relative importance of purchased services has increased. A major limiting factor on purchasing is the extent to which voluntary hospitals are willing to care for patients who have passed through the acute phase of illness.

The categorical approach limits, but does not preclude, the application of broad criteria for allocating functions between the federal government and the states and localities. Certain functions of government must be national in scope. Included are defense, which is not geographically divisible, and functions in which large economies or diseconomies accrue to persons outside the areas in which the functions are carried out, such as radio or television. Stigler would locate other functions locally and help finance them with federal grants-in-aid that do not attach controls [145, pp. 218-19].

In theory there is no reason why the Veterans Administration could not purchase psychiatric services for its beneficiaries from the state hospitals. Such an arrangement is not practicable, however, as long as the quality of care in Veterans Administration hospitals is superior [64c, p. 45].

The improvement in quality of care achieved in the Veterans Administration hospitals after World War II is a remarkable development in public administration as well as in the provision of health services. It was accomplished through the establishment of strong residency training programs in a variety of medical specialties, with the close cooperation of the deans and faculties of medical schools.

This development is in marked contrast to trends in municipal hospitals, among which hospitals not staffed by medical schools have found increasing difficulty in sustaining high quality performance. One reason is faulty administrative and budgetary procedures. The major reason, however, is their increasing inability to attract young practitioners to the attending staffs. A generation ago staff appointments to municipal hospitals were prized and sought after. The writer inquired in some detail into the drastic transformation in one large city and found a number of reasons for it. Of utmost importance are the changes in preparation for specialty practice from apprenticeship to residency training and the new economic pressures and opportunities confronting young physicians [174, pp. 155–57]. The result is that, even when a physician serves on the attending staff of a municipal hospital, he visits less often than formerly and stays a shorter period.

In sum, a government hospital does not bear the taint of profits or the profit motive [34, p. 375]. In its favor is the pursuit of a worthy purpose, that of serving the sick and dependent poor. Its defects, perhaps ineradicable in the eyes of some, pertain to inefficiency of operation by a bureaucracy subject to political pressures. One accepts deficiencies in the comforts, amenities, and courtesies afforded to patients who do not pay for their care. It is expected, however, that the quality of care would be high in an institution that is the site of medical education and medical research. Failure to realize this expectation has aroused serious concern.

Relative Shares

The proprietary form of hospital organization is apparently not acceptable, and the government hospital, especially at the local level, suffers from certain deficiencies. As a result, the voluntary form of organization enjoys a favored position. The advantage of the voluntary hospital over the municipal hospital has widened, as noted above, with respect to the recruitment of attending staff. A similar gap has appeared and widened in the respective abilities to attract house staff, nursing personnel, and administrators. Finally, although local government may have demonstrated the superior ability to build new hospitals in the postwar period, its record in maintaining the physical plant is poorer [174, pp. 260–62].

The proportion of total facilities owned by government would be smaller than it is, were it not for the operation of several factors. The presence of government hospitals frequently leads to the application of a more liberal set of criteria of eligibility for free care than otherwise and, therefore, to an increase in the size of the government system. Other factors have to do with teaching programs. For example, once Veterans Administration hospitals exist, they cannot confine themselves to caring for patients with service-connected disabilities even if this was the original intention. To exclude patients who do not have service-connected disabilities would impair the care of patients who do, for the conduct of effective teaching programs depends on the availability of a wide variety of patients to serve as clinical material. Another consideration is the inability of government hospitals to be as selective in admitting patients as other hospitals. To achieve a given level of activity in the hospital—and, equivalently, to conduct a teaching program of given size—it is necessary to maintain a larger census of patients. Still another factor is the concentration of teaching in the ward service.

Ultimately the pattern of hospital ownership is determined by the capability of the voluntary system to raise funds for capital purposes. Owing to the highly specialized functions of the hospital, as well as to the unfavorable repercussions that would result from foreclosing a mortgage on a voluntary institution, financing of construction in voluntary hospitals has historically relied on philanthropic contributions for this purpose and, to a lesser extent, on surplus income from current operations. Granting of mortgages to liquidate construction loans became feasible from the lender's standpoint when city-wide or area-wide sectarian federations agreed to underwrite a member hospital's mortgage or to draft on its behalf a letter of credit. The latter has become an accepted mode of procedure in completing that section of the application for a federal grant under the Hill-Burton program that calls for proof of the applicant's ability to meet the estimated total cost of the proposed project. Assumption of a mortgage became practicable from the borrower's standpoint when third party purchasers (Blue Cross and government) agreed to include an allowance for depreciation and interest cost in their rates of payment. (For convenience and as built-in protection against inflation, this allowance is frequently calculated as a surcharge on patient day cost rather than as a percentage of capital investment.) Lest these payments be dissipated on expenditures for current purposes, the hospital is often required to fund the depreciation allowance, that is, to set it aside and apply it only to approved capital purposes. No such requirement is, of course, imposed on business concerns.

In contemplating expansion a voluntary hospital seldom engages in a calculation of cost and benefit due to capital expenditures. Except for the effort involved in raising capital funds, the hospital acts as if capital had a zero price [176, p. 213].

D. SOME IMPLICATIONS FOR POLICY

By drawing on the analyses presented in this chapter and, in addition, on certain conclusions regarding the demand for hospital care, it is possible to derive some implications for policy.

This section deals with three areas of hospital policy: pricing, staffing, and building.

Pricing

It is frequently stated that hospital care is sold at cost and that the price charged for it reflects cost rather than demand [159, p. 35]. (Cost refers here to average unit cost.) Hospitals advocate reimbursement at cost as a matter of principle [91, p. 145].

Payment at average cost. Charging at average unit cost poses several difficulties. Implicit is the notion that the average cost of a unit of service can be calculated. That is not possible, however, when two or more goods are produced together. Each has separate, identifiable differential or marginal costs, but their joint costs cannot be disentangled in order to determine the respective average unit costs [43a, p. 307; 108, p. 359]. (It is recognized, of course, that a cost accounting procedure that cannot yield an average cost figure as a basis for pricing can yield allocations of cost among departments that facilitate managerial control.)

Moreover, cost alone cannot determine price. It is absolutely necessary to take cognizance of demand as well. One way to do this is to attribute different "revenue ratios" to the private, semi-private, and ward accommodations, in accordance with their respective capacities to raise income. This method was incorporated in a recent revision of the Blue Cross payment formula in the New York City area.

Even if the problem of multiple products is solved (by calculating average patient day cost for the hospital as a whole, on the assumption that the costs of education and research have been removed), other difficulties remain. For example, what are the elements of reimbursable cost? If cost is a historical datum recorded in books of account, how can provision be made for financing new, developmental programs? Until recently a hospital could not demonstrate new programs or expand existing ones unless it had access to other sources of funds.

Reimbursement at the full cost of each individual institution may create disincentives to efficient operation. This is aggravated by the fact that the insurance plans or government departments that pay for care do not attempt to influence the destination of patients. The share of the market accruing to a hospital is substantially independent of the level of its cost (and price).

Charging at marginal cost. Beyond these difficulties, revealed by experience, is the reluctance of many economists to accept pricing at average cost. This rule fails to meet the optimum conditions for economic equilibrium (any departure from this position signifying a loss in economic welfare). According to theory, pricing at average cost is not a sound policy in the short run and is the correct policy in the long run under competitive conditions only because average cost coincides with marginal cost.

It is true, of course, that the voluntary hospital is not a business enterprise. The pursuit of maximum profits is not its guiding principle. It has been postulated that a voluntary hospital aims to maximize the welfare of society by serving as many patients as possible, subject to certain constraints. One is that the size of its deficit cannot exceed specified limits. In the absence of income from philanthropy, this condition states that total revenues must equal total expenditures at the volume of services that will be sold [89, pp. 44, 53]. Another constraint is that the quality of care rendered should be at least adequate and the best attainable for the amount of money spent [176, p. 212]. (Sometimes there appears to be a conflict in goals between a hospital's administration and its house staff. The former aims to maintain a high average daily census, while the latter aims to admit the largest possible number of acutely ill patients. To achieve the latter, it may be necessary to maintain a reserve of vacant beds.)

Starting from these premises Feldstein proceeded to formulate criteria of pricing by a voluntary hospital. It will be recalled that the hospital's marginal cost is below average cost. To price the product at marginal cost would not recover total cost and would result in a deficit. It is necessary that price exceed marginal cost, unless funds are forthcoming from an external source. However, the aim is only to recover costs, not to maximize net revenue. Therefore, price need not be raised to the point where marginal revenue (the revenue derived from selling an additional unit of output, taking into account the reduction in price of all preceding units when competition is less than perfect) equals marginal cost. An intermediate policy is most likely to be adopted [121, pp. 65–66].

Feldstein's conclusion regarding a reasonable pricing policy by a voluntary hospital is similar to Smithies' recommendation of an appropriate pricing policy for government enterprise. Contrary to the view held by many economists, he objects to setting price at marginal cost (when it is below average cost) on the ground that the deficits of one government program compete with the revenue requirements of other programs, such as education, that cannot be financed by fees [41, p. 199]. Bator has pointed out that it is possible for an economy to suffer from greater inefficiencies than departures from marginal cost pricing. Although he approves of the general rule that prices be set at marginal cost, he would not adhere to it rigidly [56, p. 112].

If price were set at or near marginal cost, how would the resulting deficit be financed? One solution is to institute a separate charge for the hospital's stand-by service [1, p. 296]. Another would be to arrange for subsidies from tax funds or philanthropic contributions [205, p. 11]. To relate the amount of subsidy to the size of deficit or even to the amount of fixed cost in a hospital is, however, to invite inflation of expenditures [34, p. 378]. It helps to bring the amount of fixed cost outside the hospital's influence.

When the price of a product is set too low (below marginal cost in this context), it ceases to discharge effectively one of its important functions, namely, that of a rationing mechanism for equating the quantities taken and offered in a market [34, p. 403]. It becomes necessary to resort to supplementary non-financial devices. Some of these devices are: applying a means test; screening hospital admissions for good teaching material; maintaining long waiting lists for elective admissions; imposing the discomfort of queues in outpatient departments [34, pp. 358–62; 81, p. 347].

Variable pricing. Following up on a recommendation that frequently recurs, Feldstein inquired whether variable pricing might cope with fluctuations in the demand for hospital service. He concluded against a policy of charging lower prices on weekends (and holidays) than in the middle of the week. Feldstein's reasons follow, two pertaining to the price elasticity of the supply curve and two to that of the demand curve.

It may be that short-run marginal cost would not differ appreciably between peak load and off-peak load, if cognizance were taken of premium pay to hospital employees for working other than a regular shift. It may also be that the physician would charge extra for his sacrifice of leisure, thereby offsetting any reduction in the hospital bill. On the demand side, the problem is that under health insurance the patient's marginal outlay for going to the hospital is zero or negligible. In addition, since patients are apparently not knowledgeable about hospital costs and charges [121, pp. 71–73], the demand for hospital care is not likely to be responsive to variations in price.

Automatic payments formula. The writer employed the analysis of factors contributing to the rise in hospital cost in an attempt to explain the failure of a ten-year old Blue Cross reimbursement formula. When adopted in 1948, this formula received universal acclaim, for it automatically provided for a quarterly adjustment of the rate of payment to individual hospitals in accordance with the movement of certain price indexes; the size of the adjustment could not be influenced by the individual hospital; the formula eliminated protracted negotiations between Blue Cross and the hospitals; and it seemed to assure uniform and equitable treatment of all concerned.

Although the formula was applied with flexibility, it was not tenable and had to be abandoned. Its tacit assumption was that the early postwar increase in hospital cost represented a one-time catching up with wages and working conditions in other industries. A further increase in hospital cost was not expected in the absence of inflation in the economy. True, patient day cost may increase in an individual hospital, but only because of a substantial change in the scope of its program. For this purpose an adjustment outside the formula was allowed. The continued rise in hospital cost due to a relative lag in productivity was not anticipated, nor the increased cost of educational programs [132, pp. 243–44].

Staffing

The analysis of cost increases served as a point of departure for the writer's exploration of certain aspects of staffing.

Hospitals have responded to continuing pressures toward higher cost partly by acceding to them and partly by containing them. The principal means of containment is to reduce the qualifications established for certain positions. One result is that hospitals hire employees who cannot be used with flexibility or trusted to work without close supervision.

In a personal service industry it is difficult to exercise effective supervision, since standards of output are not easily set. It would be more efficient to hire persons who know their jobs, require little supervision, and may be held responsible for their performance. Indeed, one student believes that this policy is the factor chiefly responsible for the much lower staffing ratio in hospitals in Sweden than in the United States [135, p. 35].

Flexibility in using hospital personnel is desirable. Flagle and his associates found that significant gains in efficiency (reduction in length of queues) can be achieved in the clinic of a hospital if clerical and administrative personnel are assigned more than a single task [123, p. 39]. If so, employees must be hired with higher initial qualifications and greater training potential than are required to perform one task. The question is whether the relative wages of the two categories of personnel would justify the substitution of the former for the latter.

Thompson and his colleagues have generalized Flagle's finding as follows: "The most efficient way to provide any service for random arrivals who require a service for varying periods of time is to have the service performed in one place and, if possible, by one person. The assembly line method, where the total service is split among many persons and is performed in different locations, is efficient only when strict scheduling is possible" [184, p. 78]. In other words, there are limits to the advantages of division of labor. One of them is when strict scheduling cannot be observed. Another is when tasks require coordination of a delicate or complicated variety. In the latter case the loss arising from nonspecialization is offset by the gains achieved through coordination [43b, p. 140].

Building

Owing to the low ratio of marginal to average cost in the short run, vacant beds are costly. To the extent that the beds are vacant unnecessarily, the cost of operating them represents a waste.

Owing to daily fluctuations in admissions and the segregation of patients by sex (and perhaps also according to other criteria, such as diagnostic condition), a hospital is not expected to maintain an average occupancy rate of 100 percent. For many years hospital planners set the optimum rate of occupancy at 80 percent [171, p. 29], but the current consensus revolves around 85 percent [154, p. 58; 187, p. 25].

A penalty in extra vacant beds is sometimes accepted, if the additional beds comprise a service that is considered essential to the rounding out of a hospital. (This is another example of an external benefit.) Thus, an obstetrical service may be valued for its contribution to the development of the pediatric and the gynecological services, both for teaching and for patient care. It is easier to recruit interns for a self-sufficient hospital that has no need to arrange affiliations with other hospitals. Such a hospital also finds it easier to attract attending staff in the medical specialties, because they can be included in a larger, more complete network of patient referrals.

VI. ORGANIZATION, COORDINATION, AND REGULATION

It would seem worth-while to explore certain aspects of organization and coordination in the health and medical care field. Although solo practice is the most common form of medical practice in this country, the group practice form of organization has received extensive treatment in the literature and will be discussed in Section A. In Chapters IV and V we have considered the supply of physicians and of hospital services, and Section B, below, will summarize the relationships between them. It will be seen that for the most part physicians and hospitals complement and support one another; under certain conditions they serve as substitutes. Section C will deal with area-wide planning for and coordination of hospital facilities and services. Section D will deal with regulation and will raise some questions regarding the proposed public utility status for hospitals.

A. EFFECT OF GROUP PRACTICE ON THE USE OF PHYSICIANS AND HOSPITALS

The organization of physicians into groups has been advocated for many years. The argument is two-fold: (a) it results in a superior quality of medical care; and (b) it yields savings in the use of physicians and hospitals.

Quality of Care

When physicians are highly specialized it is difficult to maintain continuity of care for patients and to avoid fragmentation. Promotion of these two objectives would be facilitated if every person had a family physician to perform the screening, referral, and coordinating of medical functions, as well as to render a high proportion of all diagnostic and treatment services (estimated at 80 percent) [29, Vol. 2, p. 136]. In actuality many persons do not have a family physician and either are their own referral agents or rely on friends to recommend a specialist. In large cities the aggregate of specialty clinics maintained by an outpatient department of a hospital may come close to providing the entire range of services required by patients; however, a central point of referral and coordination is usually lacking. Even among those persons who have a family physician, there are some who seek specialists' care without his knowledge or approval. As a result, some students of medical care have come to believe that the only rational way to assure good care for a population is through the group practice of medicine in which family physicians and specialists are associated in close proximity.

The superior quality of care attributed to group practice is usually related to the advantages of an organized form of practice [42, p. 119], which include the salutary effects of peer discipline [15, p. 60], informal consultation within the staff, systematic record keeping, and continuity of care. It is said that the benefits of medical specialization are realized without the disadvantage of fragmentation of service [92, p. 677].

Little formal evidence exists to substantiate this claim in terms of the final outcome, namely, the effect on patients' health and survival. (In fairness one must state that few medical care studies have succeeded in measuring the quality of care in terms of final outcome.) A conspicuous exception are the studies of perinatal mortality (stillbirths after twenty weeks of gestation and infant deaths within thirty days of birth) conducted jointly by the Health Insurance Plan of Greater New York (HIP) and the Health Department of the City of New York [183, p. 183]. These show a significantly lower death rate for HIP subscribers than for the rest of the population. One factor was the much higher proportion of certified specialists among HIP obstetricians.

Although it is usually conceded that an organized medical group provides the superior quality of care, concern persists over the gap between promise and performance [180, p. 199]. The principal explanation of the gap is a difference in the values and norms of behavior between patients, on the one hand, and the physicians and the administrators in group health plans, on the other hand [180, p. 207]. It has been suggested that closed panel plans (under which subscribers obtain medical care from a designated medical group, paying for it in advance through premiums) are vulnerable to a deterioration in the quality of care [63, p. 81]. In this respect they appear to resemble the hospital outpatient department, which seldom achieves the standard of care of the hospital's inpatient service for the same population.

One highly regarded medical group reports an annual turn-over rate of 25 percent among its physicians. This fact indicates either an appreciable degree of dissatisfaction within the group or superior alternatives elsewhere. It also strains to an extreme what seems to be a basic presumption of organized group practice, namely, that physicians with like qualifications can take care of patients interchangeably [169, p. 45]. At least some consumers appear to be willing to pay extra for the privilege of choosing a physician, and others who belong to a group (and have paid their premium) seek care on the outside under certain circumstances or for certain purposes [169, pp. 51–52].

Efficiency in Using Physicians

It has long been held that the group practice form of organization yields a saving of physicians. The reasoning is that wasteful duplication of physicians' services is avoided, especially in diagnosis; physicians are enabled to make full use of ancillary personnel and equipment; and the idle waiting time involved in building a solo practice is eliminated.

The quantitative estimate of the saving is of the order of one third [7a, p. 266]. This figure has not been challenged for at least two reasons.

Physicians' expressions of intent notwithstanding, group practice has grown at a slow rate [7a, p. 245]. By 1959 it embraced 12,000 physicians, 6 percent of all physicians in private practice. Partly responsible has been the opposition of organized medicine to prepaid group practice, a policy only recently rescinded by the American Medical Association. Another factor is the possibility of achieving sizable financial savings by other means, such as the sharing of office expenses among physicians, which do not entail loss of autonomy [13, p. 112]. Possibly physicians see no need for the group form of organization, for today no physician practices completely alone or quite apart from colleagues.

The second reason is technical. Since most prepaid practice groups that offer comprehensive medical care to a family permit their physician members to care for patients who are not subscribers, there is no firm denominator for calculating a physician-to-population ratio.

Only recently has an economist questioned the claim that group practice yields a saving of physicians. His point is that this form of organization could hardly result in a low physician-to-population ratio if its physician members obtained all the benefits they are led to expect, including shorter and more regular hours, longer vacations, more frequent attendance at medical meetings, and occasional time off to pursue post-graduate education [202, p. 14]. (Obviously, this point does not deny the possibility of an improvement in medical care, owing to the more efficient use of the same number of physicians; this observation was made by Rashi Fein.) In adopting this view, an advisory committee to the Surgeon General observed that the physician-to-population ratios in these plans are somewhat higher than the ratio for the United States population as a whole [107, pp. 11–12].

In turn, this position has been disputed. The argument is that equal physician-to-population ratios obscure certain facts. Urban populations use more medical services than rural populations, and subscribers to prepaid group practice plans are educated and encouraged to request early and frequent medical attention [42, p. 128].   Bailey, in a study of private medical practice organization, concluded that prepaid group practice best met the four criteria of quality and efficiency that he specified [155, Chap. 4, pp. 69–75, Chap. 6, pp. 27–29]. However, his is a theoretical construct, which abstracts from attitudes and possible nonpecuniary returns from other, alternative forms of practice.

Efficiency in Using Hospitals

More recently, beginning after World War II with the steady accumulation of data, the claim has been advanced that group practice coupled with prepayment yields savings in the use of hospitals. Initially the claim was based on the routine statistics produced by several health insurance plans. Subsequently, beginning about 1955, a number of special studies of matched populations with different types of insurance for physicians' services were conducted by the Health Insurance Plan of Greater New York and others [165]. Each of these studies showed lower hospital use by subscribers to prepaid group practice plans. The differential has been put at approximately 20 percent, almost all of it attributable to a difference in the rate of hospital admission [173, p. 957].

The explanation of this finding revolves essentially about the effect of the group form of practice and the operation of group facilities, which permit hospitalization to be avoided in certain instances; and the absence of the fee-for-service principle in paying physicians, thereby eliminating a possible incentive for hospitalizing patients. The several studies did consider other explanations, among them the provision of health insurance benefits for physicians' services outside the hospital; possible failure to diagnose and treat subscribers' illnesses; and lack of access to hospital beds. Upon examination these explanations were discarded, with full realization that the evidence was not conclusive.

Other studies focus on the central role of the physician in limiting hospital use. Some students point to the authority exercised by the specialist guarding the hospital gate [178, p. 7], while others emphasize the responsibility of the general practitioner, who is the family physician, to integrate and coordinate the many services provided [168, p. 25].

In November, 1962, reports appeared on two studies of matched populations that yielded unexpected findings. In both studies, one in New York City and one in three distant sections of the country, subscribers to prepaid group practice plans reported the same rate of hospital use as subscribers to other types of health insurance plan; in every case the amount of hospital use was low [166, p. 65; 189, p. 152]. These studies served to reopen questions that had been previously regarded as settled.

In a review of these and the earlier studies, the writer asked whether the common element in low hospital use is not the exercise of controls [173, p. 963]. These can take various forms and may be carried out by salaried physicians, by subscribers confronted with financial deterrents, such as deductible clauses or co-insurance provisions, or by self-insured plans in which the members take a protective interest; or they may be enforced by the lack or inaccessibility of hospital beds. So understood, the organizational framework of group practice and the professional discipline it imposes may constitute one source of control over hospital use, as well as a vehicle for providing ambulatory services (which do not necessarily reduce hospital use). The writer also concluded that past studies have concentrated unduly on one of the components of hospital use, the rate of admission, to the neglect of the other, the average duration of patient stay [173, p. 961]. Other students have also expressed the desirability of giving greater weight to duration of stay in future studies [154, p. 57].

B. RELATIONSHIP BETWEEN THE PHYSICIAN AND THE HOSPITAL

Had the organization of hospital care in this country developed differently, that is, as a private enterprise controlled by physicians, the organization of medical practice would also have been different. Elaborate physical equipment and large numbers of ancillary personnel would have been needed in physicians' offices, and a physician could not begin practice with a modest investment in his office (of the order of $3,500) nor maintain it with one assistant or none. "Firms" and even incorporated enterprises might have been common [124, p. 261].

But the above is speculation. In fact, hospitals did develop as quasi-public enterprises under voluntary (nonprofit) or governmental auspices, and their relationship with physicians took on a distinct pattern. In this section the pattern is described, and some questions are raised concerning the effects it has produced.

Attending Staff

A noteworthy aspect of hospital management is that its key personnel, the clinicians (physicians who care for patients directly), are seldom employees. They are private practitioners who come to the hospital to use its expensive and complex facilities and equipment and to keep abreast of scientific advances. In return, they may be asked to provide free services in the ward, outpatient department, or emergency department. The medical staff of a hospital is an autonomous professional body, yet it is under the general direction of the hospital's owners. This intricate and delicate relationship is of central importance to both parties.

By custom, practicing physicians do not sit on the board of trustees of a voluntary hospital. Although the lay board is legally charged with full responsibility for the quality of medical care, it is clearly dependent on the medical staff for the discharge of the responsibility.

The physician's contact with the hospital begins early in his career. As a third- or fourth-year medical student he receives his clinical clerkship there, mostly on the ward service. He spends one year in the hospital as an intern and two and a half years, on the average, as a resident in preparation for specialty practice.

The practicing physician depends on the hospital for two types of opportunity [164, Chap. 8]. One is to continue his postgraduate education for the rest of his career. The other is to earn part of his living there. (In 1958, 40 percent of physicians' income from patients and insurance was earned in hospitals [53, p. 15].) He also receives referrals from his colleagues at the hospital, and the services of the house staff relieve him to some extent of caring for his own patients in the hospital and enable him to care for more patients outside.

The relationship between physician and hospital in this country differs from that on the European continent or in Great Britain, where specialists practice in the hospital and most general practitioners confine their practice to the outside. The British pattern antedates the radical change in medical care financing effected by the National Health Service and apparently has not been influenced by it.

It is contended that staffing a hospital with full-time specialists improves the quality of care rendered and raises efficiency of operation [178, pp. 6–7]. If hospitals in this country were to confine membership on their staffs to full specialists or diplomates certified by specialty boards, what would happen to those physicians who were considered unqualified for hospital appointment? Almost all of them would continue to practice in the community. In this instance the hospital's interest in its own performance and status is not identical with the community's broader interest in the quality of care rendered in physicians' offices and patients' homes as well as in hospitals.

But if every ethical physician is to receive a staff appointment in a voluntary or a government hospital, as some advocate, how is he to be prevented from performing diagnostic and treatment measures for which he is not competent? The answer lies in the medical staff organization of the hospital, which (under the authority of the trustees of the hospital) may legally restrict the privileges of a physician in accordance with his qualifications and experience. Sometimes the limitations imposed on performance within the hospital are extended to apply outside its walls.

In this light, the movement to establish departments of general practice in hospitals may be understood as an attempt to enhance the influence of general practitioners in matters that concern them, such as staff appointments, expansion of privileges, and promotions. A department of general practice is not a physical entity, with its own beds and facilities.

Furthermore, the denial of staff appointments to a single physician or a group of physicians by all the hospitals in an area cannot be justified. It seems reasonable to suppose that a physician who cannot qualify to work in the hospital, where supervision is available, is not qualified to practice outside the hospital, where there is none [174, p. 145]. Nor can it be logically maintained that a shortage of hospital beds exists with respect to the total number of physicians in a community. At a given time a community's hospitals will admit a certain number of patients, each of whom must be under the care of a physician. Either all physicians share in the access to the total number of beds in existence or some physicians are favored at the expense of others.

The individual hospital still faces the problem of making a selection among all actual and potential applicants, although it may owe priority of appointment to alumni from its house staff, to members of the sponsoring ethnic or religious group, and perhaps to practitioners from its immediate neighborhood. When numerous considerations enter into a decision, opportunities arise to take actions that discourage or curtail competition. The fact that most staff appointments are renewable annually puts a premium on conformity. Negro physicians are often deprived of their share of staff appointments in hospitals serving the entire community. It has been suggested that organized medicine maintains its control over the profession through the hospital [74, p. 30; 128, pp. 13–14].

Some physicians hold appointments at three or four or five hospitals, while others have none. Some duplicate appointments are courtesy appointments. (The distinction between an appointment to the attending staff and an appointment to the courtesy staff is that the former is a full-fledged appointment, combining private patient privileges and service on the ward and participation in teaching, while the latter pertains only to private patient privileges. Courtesy appointments are intended to increase the hospital's patient census, although the holder of such an appointment may have a lower priority for securing a hospital bed for his patients.)

It is difficult for a physician to make valuable contributions to several hospitals. Furthermore, competition among hospitals to cater to individual physicians may lead to an overestimate of the pressure for beds. (This possibility was originally suggested by Robert Sigmond.) The obvious remedy would be to eliminate or limit multiple staff appointments. This proposal may be unacceptable, because it entails interference with the autonomy of hospitals and physicians. Moreover, its total adoption would be unwise, for the selective duplication of staff appointments in certain medical specialties is a prerequisite to any serious attempt to coordinate services among hospitals [174, p. 326].

Full-Time Clinical Physicians

Full-time clinicians comprise a relatively small group of physicians in the hospital. Their increasing numbers are a reflection of the rising complexity of technology in medicine. Direction of a department or an educational program by a member of the voluntary attending staff is sometimes found to be unworkable, for its members cannot devote the necessary time.

Three types of appointment are made:

1. A director of medical education, full-time or part-time. This may be a young physician who has recently completed his residency training and is assigned the task of coordinating the hospital's several educational programs. His authority may not be commensurate.

2. A full-time chief of clinical service. He is in charge of his department and usually receives a salary. He may or may not have the privilege of seeing private patients. If he does, fees usually accrue to the hospital or to a special departmental fund for research. After the initial outlay his services may entail no cost to the hospital if he succeeds in attracting a sufficient volume of research grants.

3. A geographic full-time position. Its holder has his office at the hospital but derives all or most of his income from the care of private patients. Since he is obviously in economic competition with the other attending physicians, he may become a focus of dissension.

Hospitals maintain still other relationships with their physician staff members. A few sponsor or house a group practice unit. Others maintain doctors' offices for renting to members of their staff, whether on a full- or part-time basis. Still other hospitals offer some of the services of their organized home care programs to patients of private practitioners on their staff.

Ancillary Departments

Pathologists, radiologists, and anesthesiologists comprise

a special category of physicians. They do not have patients of their own, but care for those admitted by other members of the attending staff. This fact has created certain difficulties. On the one hand, a built-in clientele and monopoly power attach to the very privilege of the hospital staff appointment. The monopoly is created by the hospital when it acts to exclude competitors. The patient has neither choice nor knowledge of the specialist in question; and the hospital assumes full responsibility for the quality of his services [42, p. 82]. On the other hand, hospitals tend to charge for X-ray and laboratory services at the rates prevailing in physicians' offices in the community (in order to escape the allegation of cut-rate competition), thereby obtaining surplus earnings. When hospitals appropriate these departmental surpluses for general operating purposes, they are accused of engaging in the corporate practice of medicine, which is both illegal and unethical; and the physicians insist on securing more businesslike financial arrangements. No objection is raised to paying physicians a salary when the patients involved are poor and do not pay for their own care [156].

The hospitals maintain that they must not be turned into hotels that grant private concessions to physicians. Moreover, they do not wish to become involved in the rival jurisdictional claims of Blue Cross (hospital care insurance) and Blue Shield (physician care insurance) plans [156]. Despite the wide, earnest, and sometimes acrimonious discussion that surrounds this aspect of the physician-hospital relationship, there is no indication that hospital-specialist arrangements are being altered on a wholesale scale [42, pp. 81–82]. In New York State some pathologists and radiologists have shifted from salaried status alone toward a combination of part salary and a percentage of departmental revenue [186, p. 158].

C. PLANNING AND COORDINATING HOSPITAL CARE

In the hospital industry, unlike most other areas of economic activity in this country, the 1960s have witnessed a widespread movement toward external planning and coordination. Absence of coordination in hospital facilities and services is seen as the "face of anarchy" and as evidence of the lack of any system.

Area-wide Planning

Experts, officials, and the public expect that planning and coordination will reduce the cost of hospital care or at least curtail its rise in the future. Control over cost will be accomplished by (a) limiting the number of beds; (b) avoiding (and eliminating) duplication of expensive facilities that are rarely used or require for operation a large, highly trained staff—cobalt radiation therapy and heart surgery are ubiquitous examples; and (c) using the costly hospital bed to maximum advantage by establishing cheaper substitute facilities and services in adequate numbers.

As for the last of these measures, a cautionary note may be in order. Average patient day cost in a hospital is the weighted average of the costs of caring for patients with different degrees of illness and, therefore, different (heavy, medium, and low) requirements for service.

The economic bases of the drive to control and limit the number of hospital beds are (a) the low proportion of marginal to average patient day cost in the short run, which makes a vacant bed costly; (b) the possible effect of the supply of beds on hospital use, which, if confirmed, would indicate that attempts to fill gaps in hospital care will come to nought and can only result in incessant increases in total expenditures; and (c) random fluctuations in admissions to short-term hospitals, which render costly the segregation of any category of patients and the specialization of facilities of small size.

Avoiding Vacant Beds

Most formulas for estimating hospital bed requirements reflect the belief that a simple and one-way relationship exists between hospital use and a population's need. With admissions or patient days serving as the dependent variable, early formulas commonly employed size of population and the death rate as the independent variables [162, pp. 293–95; 171, p. 29]. The death rate was intended to represent the age composition of a population, with a high death rate reflecting a high proportion of aged. It is as if illness and the use of medical services were exclusively biological phenomena, which they are not [8, p. 233].

In recent years consideration has been given to including additional demographic and socioeconomic variables in calculating a population's hospital bed requirements, such as marital status, health insurance, educational level, race. The respective weights of the several factors are not yet sufficiently well established to permit their incorporation in a formula. For example, some students attach a great deal of importance to marital status and see it as explaining much of the extra hospital use usually associated with aging [52, p. 71]. There is an indication that being married may be associated with higher hospital use among young people and with lower use among old people [158, p. 736]. Rosenthal found that hospital use is significantly correlated with marital status but not with age [181, pp. 33, 40]. In explanation he suggests that possibly geographic areas with a high proportion of aged contain large numbers of alternative facilities, such as nursing homes [181, p. 34]. Another possibility is that the correlation between old age and (low) income may mask other relationships. Since a low income area is likely to contain relatively few hospital beds, its aged population may use a disproportionately large share of a given bed capacity.

For the time being, present use remains the best indicator of future use [167, p. 43; 187, p. 23]. In England planners make an allowance for a change in the size of the waiting list. The reliability of waiting lists has been questioned [152, pp. 38–39; 172, pp. 39–40].

A difficult step in the planning process is the delineation of boundaries for planning areas. In a large city it is misleading to draw hard and fast lines between the area served by one hospital and that served by another.

Another difficulty in planning pertains to the choice between need and demand as a basis for recommending in favor of, or against, the building of beds. A hospital that is "needed" but not used is still a white elephant. There is a tendency for persons associated with hospitals, both professionals and volunteers, to set a high value on hospital care and perhaps an even higher one on hospital buildings. One of the lessons economics teaches, it has been well said, is that single aims have their (high) price [160, p. 54].

It is also necessary to deal with the diversity of hospital ownership. Suppose that the net balance between the number of beds required and that available in an area shows a certain size of deficit, and it is recommended that this number of beds be built. If the recommendation is adopted and carried out, over-building can still ensue. The reason is that the count of available beds includes only beds in suitable buildings. The hospital that is requested to build may not be the same as the hospital that owns unsuitable facilities. If the latter's beds continue in operation, what is intended as a replacement may turn out to be an expansion.

As Dewhurst discovered, forecasting the population of the United States only seven years ahead can be a chastening experience [7b, p. 73]. Forecasting population for small areas is a particularly hazardous undertaking, and it is often avoided by planners. (Examples are the state hospital plans prepared under the Hill-Burton program and the British studies of bed requirements [152, p. 84].) Yet a projection of bed requirements can be no better than the population base to which the probable rate of hospital use is applied.

Given also the prospect of further technological changes, it is almost certain that some of the most carefully prepared plans will prove to be faulty. A proper goal is to minimize the losses resulting from mistaken forecasts.

Influence of Supply on Use

A research finding that carries drastic implications for policy is that the supply of and demand for hospital services are not independent forces, for the very availability of hospital beds promotes their use. If this proposition is true, it means that no number of beds (within the range of observed experience) will suffice. Rather than filling an existing need, an increase in capacity serves to raise demand (shift the demand curve to the right). Granted that there are no absolute standards of appropriate hospital use [153, p. 3] and the possibility (but by no means certainty) that in some areas there may be more persons outside the hospital who require its services than persons inside who do not, it is at least equally true that hospital care is not in itself a desirable object of consumption, which is to be encouraged.

The evidence presented to date on the relationship between increased bed supply and use is not conclusive. We have impressions from experience and from statistical analysis. The controversy is colored by the implication that use lifted by the influence of supply incorporates a substantial element of overuse or abuse.

Roemer is generally credited with having offered the first formal statement of the proposition that the more hospital beds, the more patient days in the hospital. His proof consisted of two parts. First, a high degree of correlation exists between the number of short-term hospital beds in an area (state or county) and average patient census, and there is virtually no association between the supply of beds and the rate of occupancy [182, pp. 72–73]. The corollary is that general hospital beds are occupied at approximately the same rate, regardless of the ratio of beds to population. Second, in a county in upstate New York a new hospital of 200 beds was built, representing an expansion in bed supply of 42 percent, and within three years patient days had increased 28 percent. There were no other changes in the community that might account for the rise in hospital use [179, p. 38].

Rosenthal has challenged Roemer's conclusions on several grounds: (a) Roemer's state-wide data show a wide range in rates of occupancy; (b) the range is only slightly reduced when the (downward) effect of small size is allowed for; and (c) an association between high use of hospital beds and high levels of supply is not a sufficient basis for concluding that an increase in supply creates demand. It may be that hospitals are built where demand exists [181, pp. 62, 63, 66]. Supply does not just appear; it arises in response to pressures, one of which could be the demand for facilities. Rosenthal found that, when the variables associated with both supply and demand are held constant, higher levels of demand are associated with greater pressure on facilities and higher levels of supply with lesser pressure on facilities [181, pp. 67, 69].

In the writer's opinion Rosenthal has demonstrated that the association between supply and use is not one to one. However, Roemer does not make so precise a claim. The fact is that the forces impinging on the supply of beds and on the demand for hospital care are by no means identical. For example, a voluntary hospital may decide to expand when it receives a donation or bequest. The decision when and where to build a government hospital may rest on the relative political influence of a councilman. Funds for building may be more readily available for some purposes than for others, so that research buildings receive priority over educational or patient care buildings, inpatient buildings over outpatient buildings, and new construction over remodeling an existing building.

Today most students of hospital care believe that for the purpose of policy formulation (or planning) it is best to assume that, under prevailing conditions (particularly payment by third parties for substantial volumes of hospital care), the supply of beds does influence use [151, p. 33; 168, p. 20; 177, Vol. 2, p. 823]. A few consider the relationship one of association, not of causality [167, p. 42]. Only Airth and Newell in England have squarely faced Rosenthal's third point and concluded that the difference in hospital use between their two areas of study can be attributed only to a difference in available beds [152, p. 75].

As long as the primary risk of additional hospital building was the high cost of a vacant bed (due to the high proportion of fixed to total cost), each institution was confronted by a financial deterrent. When the principal danger is unnecessary use, the interests of the individual institution and of society may diverge. As a result, some students of hospital care have come to advocate that the total number of beds in an area be limited and, therefore, that hospital building be controlled [159, pp. 108–9; 174, p. 524].

Cost of Variation in Patient Census

A network of large hospitals may be expected to operate at a higher average rate of occupancy than a network of small hospitals and, therefore, to be able to accommodate a given average daily census with fewer beds. The proof is frequently advanced in terms of the Poisson statistical distribution [162, p. 279]. However, not all services of the hospital conform to the requirements of this distribution, namely, random behavior of admissions and only a small proportion of the population requiring hospitalization at a given time [157, p. 78]. Undoubtedly the maternity service conforms, with minor adjustment for induced labor; while surgery, with an appreciable proportion of elective admissions, may not.

Long studied the implications of variable demand by analyzing patient data for fourteen hospitals in the Pittsburgh area. (The data had been originally collected for another purpose.) His point of departure is the statistical proof that the average daily census for a consolidated group of hospitals is more stable (has a lower coefficient of variation) than that for the sum of several hospitals acting independently [176, draft]. An exception to this generalization, and the only one, would be the presence of perfect positive correlation among the census of the several hospitals. In actuality, peak patient loads seldom occur simultaneously in every hospital [175a, p. 61]. Accordingly, fewer beds are required to furnish a given level of protection if hospitals cooperate than if they act independently.

As the concern over rising hospital cost has mounted and medical technology has become more specialized and more complex, hospitals of large size have seemed to yield such large gains in efficiency that the very desirability of distributing hospital beds in relation to the distribution of population (residence of patients) has come to be challenged. It is proposed that the minimum size of a hospital in a metropolitan area be 200 beds [187, p. 28] or perhaps 300 [151, p. 33]. Preliminary results by Coughlin and Isard point to an optimum size of 700 beds and higher. However, their figures are based on scale curves (showing variation of unit cost with size of activity), that were derived hypothetically from replies to questions asked of hospital department heads [163a, pp. 24–25].

Others affirm that due consideration of travel distance for

patients and visitors may preclude building hospitals of the most efficient size [121, p. 64; 152, p. 24]. To achieve the best results one should aim to balance expressly the inconvenience and other costs of additional travel time to a small number of larger hospitals against the alleged benefits in quality of care and economy of operation, and to compare the result with the costs and benefits of a network of more and smaller hospitals. It is not enough to say that one arrangement costs less than or is superior to another; the question is by how much [153, p. 5]. Coughlin and Isard found that for all concerned transportation costs to and from a hospital amounted to 19 percent of its operating costs [163b, p. 38]; this figure may be on the low side, since it is based on distance without regard for travel time.

Long attempted to measure the benefits derived from some degree of flexibility within an institution plus a modest degree of interhospital cooperation in admitting patients. From the Pittsburgh data he estimated the gains from three devices, each employed on a limited scale: "swing" beds (beds that could be used on different specialty services, depending upon need), an average of three per hospital; delaying admission of nonemergency patients for a maximum of three days; and interhospital shifting of admissions, an average of forty-two a year by each hospital. He calculated a saving in beds of 7 percent [176, p. 221]. Two thirds of the saving is attributable to the third device, which would be by far the most controversial [176, draft]. Long's number of swing beds is small, and the period of delay in admitting elective admissions altogether short.

Coordination on the modest scale envisaged above may be practicable. More extensive coordination is hindered by the prevailing pattern of ownership. There is little or no intercourse between proprietary hospitals and the others, and differences in clientele preclude across-the-board coordination between voluntary and municipal hospitals. There is also a distinct difference in their respective abilities to screen admissions selectively.

Nonprofit activity usually means activity by local volunteers. Their interests are not readily transferable from one geographic area to another.

Much of the discussion of area-wide coordination is couched in terms of the short-term hospital, as is the work on planning. Yet acute hospitalized illness is episodic, and good care is not too dependent on coordination among institutions and between the institution and the home. In long-term care such coordination is essential.

Although sectarian ownership precludes merger, it does not hinder coordination among short-term hospitals under voluntary auspices. Indeed, there need be no relationship between ownership and the religious composition of patients. Sectarian ownership is also an important feature of long-term care. Here, however, the ownership of the institution and the religious faith of its clientele are likely to coincide. Adoption of a nondiscriminatory admission policy, as required by the Hill-Burton program, is not in fact meaningful (if only because of the patients' own preferences). A person is, therefore, dependent upon the foresight and voluntary activity of his confreres for access to a long-term facility of good quality [172, p. 47].

It is premature to attempt to draw conclusions regarding the potentialities and achievements of area-wide planning for hospitals in this country. Some problems warrant attention. In studies of long-term care it is important to emphasize the time dimension, that is, the frequency with which changes occur in patients' medical condition and in their requirement for services. This frequency sets a limit to the practicability of transferring patients from one institution to another. Also to be taken into account is the difference between the criteria followed by an institution for admitting patients and those (less rigorous) for retaining them.

In examining hospital planning one is struck by the absence of a distinction between planning as the exercise of detailed controls and planning as the design and development of a framework within which social and individual interests are brought into closer accord. The first is retail regulation, of which many economists tend to be skeptical. The second is akin to the employment of broad fiscal and monetary measures and incentives to promote specified policy objectives.

D. REGULATION

The health and medical care industry is not the domain of free enterprise. The case for intervention by government or by philanthropy in financing health and medical services has been elaborated in Chapter III, Section B. Criteria for production by government or by nonprofit organizations were discussed in Chapter V, Section C. This section deals with intervention through regulation for the purpose of achieving diverse objectives, such as the assuring of quality of care or the avoidance of economic waste.

Quality of Care

A major reason for attempting to regulate an economic activity is consumer ignorance. When the consumer is unable to appraise the usefulness of a product, society cannot rely on the rule of *caveat emptor* (let the buyer beware) [161, pp. 19, 127]. Drugs are a good example today of supervision by government. Licensure of physicians, dentists, nurses, and other personnel is a more traditional device for assuring the quality of practitioners, in terms of both intellectual attainment and integrity of character. When an organized profession participates in the process of licensure, it may be actuated by additional considerations, including concern over the economic status of members already in the profession [11, pp. 159-61; 128, p. 10]. In today's world the staff organization of the hospital—its rules and committees—is still another means for controlling the conduct of the medical profession.

The consumer may have the requisite knowledge but fail to act on it. If he is unable to do so, government action can help give effect to the judgment of individuals by concert, in John Stuart Mill's language. Sometimes the individual chooses not to act on the information in his possession. To protect society against communicable disease requires compulsory action, because one or two dissenters could undo the actions of all others [58, pp. 155-56]. Willing or not, the individual cannot be allowed to escape a quarantine invoked as a public health measure [24, p. 790]. Coercion would seem to be particularly warranted when promptness of compliance is essential. Regulation is one way to intervene on the supply side when private and social costs diverge, as in attempting to control smoke nuisance or to prevent water pollution.

Government action does not always entail enforcement measures. Sometimes it is possible to encourage compliance by reducing the extra (marginal) cost of the desired action to zero, or by subsidizing it [229, p. 27]. Government can also move to reduce certain undesirable types of consumption by employing the tax mechanism as a sumptuary device. In light of current knowledge an example might be the imposition of a heavy tax on cigarettes and of a lighter tax on liquor.

Employed as an educational tool, government regulation can serve to improve the level of performance. The education of owners of hospitals or nursing homes is helpful when the total volume of facilities is in short supply and the drastic penalty of closing deficient facilities is not available; or when an activity is expanding rapidly and the inexperienced persons trying to provide the service require assistance. Regulation through education is particularly appropriate in the performance of professional services, for which standards are complex and diverse. There is no reason why regulation by government should differ in content or form from accreditation (or approval) by voluntary (including professional) organizations.

The effectiveness of regulation depends largely on the quality of inspection. Sometimes the educational objective is emphasized over that of securing compliance with the letter of the law. Sometimes nurse or lay inspectors of hospitals are employed. Since they do not speak with the same authority as physicians, they may not be equally effective. Frequently several inspectors descend upon an institution, and orders are repeated or even countermanded. Seldom do we encounter a team of inspectors composed of recognized experts in several disciplines. When an agency with operating functions also performs regulatory functions, it may be tempted to apply less stringent criteria to its own institutions than to others.

Public Utility Status

It has been proposed that hospitals be accorded public utility status [159, pp. 108-9]. (It is interesting that as long ago as 1946 Basil McLean referred to the increasing acceptance of the hospital as a public utility.) The objective is to control and limit the supply of hospital facilities.

Public utility regulation is common in water, gas, electricity, and telephone—activities in which a large capital investment is required for developing a delivery system. If two or more suppliers rendered service in the same geographic area, there would be unnecessary duplication of facilities. A single supplier provides a less costly service because the quantity of services taken by any one household is small relative to the feasible capacity of the entire delivery system [34, p. 360]. Accordingly, society creates a legal monopoly. The state issues a certificate of necessity authorizing the provision of services and, in return, exacts a limitation on charges (and profits) and a commitment to adhere to certain standards of performance.

In all these fields the state restricts the number of firms. There is no restriction, however, on the size of the investment undertaken by a firm endowed with public utility status. How much and when to invest is determined by the firm's best business judgment, provided that it meets the standard of adequacy of service. Although a ceiling is set on the rate of return on investment, there is no guarantee that the schedule of charges prescribed by the regulatory authority will yield a given rate of profit. If a state agency were to regulate the size of individual hospitals, as well as the number of hospitals, it would be embarking on a significant departure from the traditional public utility concept.

Perhaps the public utility concept or an analogous form of legal control would be more congenial to the public if the bulk of hospital care were furnished by proprietary institutions. It is difficult to get legislators to enact restrictions on voluntary agencies whose sole mission is to serve the public interest out of love of mankind. Rather, the tendency is to extend exemptions, either from taxes or from labor laws governing relations between employers and employees or establishing minimum wages.

The public utility analogy also entails some degree of over-simplification. The delivery system of a single water company or electric company can conveniently serve a large geographic area. This is not true of hospitals. The notion that a hospital is—or should be—a community (or even neighborhood) institution cannot be lightly dismissed. One must consider travel time for patients and for visitors, as well as for physicians practicing in the community. The public may be willing to pay a price for more convenient access to hospitals, or it may not; we do not know.

In order to apply to hospitals, the public utility concept requires modification. True, there is widespread agreement that the number of hospital beds in an area must be limited. This objective can be served by a policy of deliberate speed in reviewing requests for the approval of construction projects.

VII. SELECTED PROBLEMS

Economists have studied several fields that do not fit easily into the framework of supply and demand analysis adopted for this monograph. One such field is medical prices, which is largely a problem of measurement and statistical deflation (converting current dollars into constant dollars by allowing for the rise in prices). Estimates of changes in productivity belong in this field (Section A). Another field, that of how much a nation can afford to spend on health and medical care, is largely a matter of value judgments; what some economists have said on this subject will be briefly presented in Section C. Finally, there is the currently active field of cost and benefit calculation. Some of the issues involved are implicit in the preceding chapters. However, owing in large part to our concern with the sources of economic growth, the study of investment in human resources has become a rapidly expanding field of activity for economists. It would seem useful to present an integrated discussion of this subject in the context of evaluation of health and medical care programs (Section B).

A. APPLICATIONS OF THE MEDICAL CARE PRICE INDEX

A price index is a measure of the change in price between two years for a given basket of goods. It serves as a device for dividing changes in expenditures into two (or more) components, those due to price and those due to real output. There is no perfectly satisfactory method for accomplishing this separation, because the prices and outputs of all goods do not change in the same proportion. Consumers adjust their consumption, whenever possible, in response to changes in the relative prices of goods and services, substituting cheaper items for those that have become more expensive [226, p. 52]. An index computed by pricing in both years the basket of goods bought in the base year differs from that computed by pricing in both years the basket bought in the terminal year. This is the general theoretical problem of index numbers [190, p. 77]; it does not pose special difficulties when applied to the health and medical care industry.

Data on retail prices are compiled by the U.S. Bureau of Labor Statistics for its Consumer Price Index. These data suffer from certain limitations. Thus, the data pertain to the expenditures of working class and clerical families in certain large cities; we do not know how well they represent the prices facing rural families or well-to-do and poor families in cities. Most economists believe that the Index lags in introducing new products and makes inadequate allowance for changes in quality. Despite the lack of empirical evidence, a majority of economists believe that most changes in the quality of medical care, though not all, represent improvements [226, p. 35]. If so, the Index overstates the rise in medical care prices.

The Consumer Price Index comprises eight major categories, of which medical care is one. In 1958 medical care accounted for 5.4 percent of the total weights. The medical care component consists, in turn, of 18 items that are presumed to be representative of all medical goods and services [42, pp. 192–93].

The medical care component has certain limitations of its own. It may be helpful to discuss these special limitations within the context of the purposes for which the data are employed.

Measuring Changes in Productivity

Through indirect methods a number of calculations have been made of changes-in the productivity of physicians and hospitals.

Physicians. In the late 1940s and early 1950s, Dickinson, then with the American Medical Association, applied the indirect method to physicians. In his early writings he took cognizance of the technical limitations of his procedure. In later writings there developed a tendency to present the numerical results without qualification. His final estimates of the productivity gain per physician achieved in the decade 1940–50 ranged between one third [117, p. 7] and one half [198, p. 19].

Dickinson calculated productivity by the following method: Each year he divided consumer expenditures for physicians (as estimated by the National Income Division of the U.S. Department of Commerce) by the physician price component of the Consumer Price Index. He then divided the quotient by the number of physicians in independent private practice. The result was adjusted (implicitly) to allow for the rise in the percentage of physicians' charges collected and, secondarily, for the decline in the volume of free care [196, p. 17]. The downward adjustment was warranted, for expenditures had increased without a commensurate increase in the production of services. Dickinson was also concerned over the lack of comparability in coverage between the numerator (consumer expenditures, a nationwide aggregate) and the denominator (the retail price index for families of city wage earners and clerical workers with moderate income) [198, p. 19]. The direction of bias was unknown, however.

A close examination of the data suggests several qualifications. These pertain to the necessary distinction between an increase in productivity and improved utilization of existing capacity.

a. The postwar rise in output by physicians reflects longer hours of work and increased exertion on their part, as well as higher productivity [155, Chap. 2, p. 53].

b. The advent of prosperity in the 1940s meant that young physicians developed a practice at an earlier stage in their careers. This represents an element of improved utilization, which is not the same as an increase in productivity (capacity to produce) per physician.

c. As the pipeline for graduate medical education lengthens, the age distribution of practicing physicians shifts upward. Older physicians are better established in practice and, on the average, produce more services (up to a point).

Other qualifications pertain to the behavior of physicians' fees and incomes.

a. In times of prosperity more people receive higher incomes, and more of them are affected by the sliding scale of charges.   The Consumer Price Index does not reflect these shifts.

b. In the base year, 1940, the collection ratio for physicians' income was subject to a transitional effect, as the economy passed from depression to prosperity. The implication of an improvement in the ratio between 1940 and 1950 is to call for a downward adjustment in the calculated gain in productivity during the decade. The implication of an overstatement in the collection ratio in the base year over the preceding year, however, is that the calculated improvement in collections during the decade is understated. If so, the downward adjustment applied to the calculated gain in productivity between 1940 and 1950 is too small.

c. Over the years the reporting of physicians' incomes to the Internal Revenue Service has probably improved. If so, the rise in average physician income is overstated.

Technical grounds have been advanced for the belief that the Consumer Price Index understates the rise in physicians' prices.

a. The sample of reporting physicians is overweighted with older practitioners, who tend to raise fees less frequently than their younger colleagues [22, p. 39].

b. Physicians practicing in the suburbs are excluded from the sample [42, p. 202]. Their fees may have risen faster than those of urban practitioners, owing to a more rapidly rising demand for medical services in the face of a lag in the supply of physicians [22, p. 39].

c. In any one city the sample of reporting physicians is small [211, p. 4]; this raises some questions regarding the reliability of the data. Moreover, a small sample cannot yield the variations in charges due to health insurance and the sliding scale [224, p. 321].

d. Most of the reported prices are fees charged by general practitioners, which are lower than those of specialists rendering the same service. In addition, the Index excludes many services performed only by specialists [224, p. 321]. It should be noted, however, that, even if the prices of the excluded procedures are higher, their rates of increase are not necessarily greater [216, p. 3].

  e. Physicians' fees reported in the Index are standard fees. Possibly these were reported as unchanged while actual, substandard fees were being raised. (This would be true if health insurance succeeded in enrolling many persons who formerly paid lower than standard fees) [63, p. 255].

Notwithstanding these questions and reservations, it seems plausible that the productivity of physicians (defined in terms of numbers of patients' visits) did in fact rise. Dickinson cited as explanatory factors the "wonder drugs" that accelerate healing, the large increase in subprofessional and unskilled helpers, improvements in transportation, and the decline in physicians' visits to the home and the expansion of services in the hospital and physician's office [198, p. 19]. In the writer's opinion, the antibiotic drugs probably represent a clear saving in physicians' time (except for infections that persist after a bacterium becomes resistant). The number of auxiliary personnel certainly increased, but part of the increase is not associated with a gain in physician productivity. Some of the work performed by technicians in hospitals is new or additional work, which is required by improved diagnostic procedures. Anesthesiology is an example of physicians serving as assistants to (or associates of) other physicians, namely, surgeons. Some of the visits to general practitioners result in a referral to a specialist, rather than in treatment. Improved transportation can scarcely be said to be a phenomenon of the 1940s; indeed, the converse is more likely as a result of the increased congestion of traffic. Concentration of patients in the hospital and in the physician's office is, of course, a real gain. This is due not only to the saving in travel time but also to the employment of more auxiliary personnel and house staff [155, Chap. 1, pp. 4–5]. Changes have also taken place in the organization of the physician's office and in his typical appointment schedule [42, p. 49].

A decade after Dickinson's studies, two sets of calculations of changes in physician productivity were performed by Garbarino. His earlier study found an annual gain of 3 percent during the postwar period ending in 1951 [202, p. 13]; this is close to Dickinson's figure. The estimate was qualified, however; it was possibly too high by one fifth, since an adjustment for improved collections was neglected [202, p. 15]. His later study reported a gain in productivity of 10 percent for the entire period 1949–54 [63, p. 47]. Garbarino concluded that Dickinson's results for the decade of the 1940s were due mostly to the effect of the war, when the utilization of physicians' capacity rose rapidly and the work week lengthened. He found little gain in productivity after World War II and none before the war when physicians' capacity was underutilized.

In his study of rates of return, Hansen states that the productivity of physicians increased at a high rate in the 1950s [126, p. 78], but offers no supporting evidence. Bailey, writing in 1963, estimates an increase in physician productivity of 3.3 percent a year during the period 1949–59, with even a higher rate for the latter part of the decade [155, Chap. 2, p. 55].

In calculating the productivity of physicians, price per visit is clearly the proper unit of account in the price index if requirements for physicians are calculated on the same basis. To calculate how much better (or worse) off the consumer is today than formerly, other units of account have been proposed.

One such unit is cost per episode of illness. In most cases, it is argued, what the consumer buys when he seeks medical care is not a variety of different medical services but treatment for whatever ails him [225, p. 136]. The task of the physician, one might say, is to cure as many ailments as possible, not to see as many patients as possible. The counterargument is that the patient does not contract with the physician for a recovery and is not sure of getting one when he buys medical care [203, p. 994].

It is appropriate to ask whether a price index per episode of illness is as meaningful when health and medical care is financed through health insurance benefits as it would be under conditions of direct, out-of-pocket payment by patients. A change in the health insurance premium reflects changes in both price and per capita use of services. Although the use of services may be in part the result of changes in morbidity, it is also the result of changes in socioeconomic conditions, medical technology, and medical practice.

Apart from the problems of measurement, doubts have been expressed whether it is worth-while to pursue further gains in physician productivity. The point is that it is undesirable to stint on the amount of time required to cultivate the physician-patient relationship, which is a key element in the provision of effective medical care [42, p. 51; 107, p. 12].

Hospitals. When consumer expenditures for hospital care are divided by the hospital component of the Consumer Price Index, the result is an estimate of the output of hospital services. The percentage increase in this estimate is far lower than that shown by data on trends in the volume of hospital services rendered (patient days and outpatient visits). One possible explanation of this discrepancy is that the Price Index overstates the increase in hospital price. Another is that data on the volume of hospital services rendered are inaccurate indicators of output.

Bost cites some evidence in support of the hypothesis that the Price Index may be too high. He believes that the content of the hospital's room and board has increased and refers to improvements in dietetics and in the standards of nursing care [193, p. 48]. The Commission on Financing Hospital Care reports a much higher rate of increase in the room rate than in charges for ancillary services [127, p. 58]; the latter are not reflected in the Price Index.

In the writer's opinion these points are not conclusive. The presence of increasing numbers of private duty nurses in hospitals indicates at least one source of possible diminution in the content of room and board. Since fewer hospitals apply inclusive rates to self-paying patients today than formerly, the room rate may represent a declining fraction of the hospital's total charges. This effect would be in addition to that attributable to the increased use of ancillary services per patient day. The average daily charge for all such services combined would furnish a more appropriate comparison with the room rate than prices per units of service. (It is worth noting that the data on use and price of ancillary services presented by the Commission on Financing Hospital Care are not mutually consistent, because they were drawn from diverse sources. When juxtaposed, they lead to the interesting—but erroneous—conclusion that a surgical patient in 1952 had two operations in the course of a single hospital stay, but only one in 1935 [127, pp. 59–60].) At one time the writer concluded from New York City data that the average daily charge for ancillary services was rising more rapidly than the room rate, as hospitals pursued a policy of reducing visible price competition. In the nation as a whole there was an increase in the proportion of ancillary to total hospital charges in the postwar period [211, p. 2].

Bost pointed out that the Consumer Price Index collects its data in large cities, where hospital costs and charges are higher than in small cities or rural areas. There is no reason to believe, however, that hospitals in large cities have experienced the greater rise in cost.

A partial explanation of the discrepancy noted by Bost occurs to the writer. The data reported by the United States Department of Commerce probably understate the true increase in consumer expenditures for hospital care. Derived largely from data on expenditures by voluntary hospitals, no allowance is made for the gap filled by income from patients as income from philanthropy declined in relative importance.

Drugs. The rapid introduction of new and modified drugs has created a problem in interpreting changes in the drug component of the Consumer Price Index. The Price Index includes a high proportion of older, less expensive drugs while physicians' prescriptions are overwhelmingly for new and high priced drugs [42, pp. 24, 96]. From this contrast many infer that the Price Index understates the true increase in drug prices [22, p. 38].

This conclusion is erroneous. A lag in incorporating new drugs into a price index means that such drugs are reported at prices lower than those at which they were originally introduced. If so, the price index will fail to reflect the drop in price that usually occurs during the first year or two of a product's life [226, p. 53]. An index that consistently underrepresents new and more costly products has an upward bias, rather than the reverse.

It has been suggested that drug companies hesitate to reduce price lest others match it [42, pp. 19, 211]. Lasagna sees so called "price fixing"˙as the result of automatically pegging the price of a new product at a price similar to that of the first drug introduced for a particular market, in order to avoid cutthroat competition; he doubts that there is collusion among firms [212, p. 145].

Allocation of Expenditures Increase among Factors

The medical care component of the Consumer Price Index has been employed in allocating an increase in expenditures among several factors. When two factors—price and quantity— are involved, an increase in expenditures between two years can be expressed as an equation in three terms.

$$\Delta (PQ) = \Delta P Q_0 + \Delta Q P_0 + \Delta P \Delta Q$$

P_0 and Q_0 represent price and quantity, respectively, in the base year; and ΔP and ΔQ represent changes in price and in quantity between the base and terminal years.

The first term in the equation pertains to the effect of price change; the second, to the effect of quantity change; and the third represents the interaction between changes in price and in quantity. The third term has the undesirable characteristic of increasing with the lengthening of the time interval [6, p. 153].

When three or more factors are involved (say, population is introduced), the equation expressing the increase in expenditures becomes longer and more calculations are required. The procedure can be simplified by substituting index numbers for the absolute figures. (The index number of a product equals the product of the index numbers of the factors.) It is then possible to calculate the contribution of each factor directly, this being expressed by its index number minus 100 [76, Appendix A].

How to treat the interaction term presents a problem in all analyses of data on long-term growth [214]. Three approaches are prevalent. Method 1: Distribute the interaction term proportionately between the price and quantity terms of the equation (this is equivalent to disregarding the interaction); Method 2: Share the interaction term equally between the other two terms of a three-term equation; and Method 3: Adopt a system of priorities. In effect, the third approach is employed when expenditures are first deflated by price; in a two-factor analysis the effect of deflation is to attribute the entire interaction term to price.

A helpful solution has been suggested by Denison [6, p. 105]. The interaction term virtually disappears when the percentage increase over a time interval is converted into an average annual rate of increase. (A compound interest table does this if the geometric mean is taken as the appropriate average.)

The following table applies Methods 1 and 3 (using index numbers) and Method 1 (using annual rates of increase) to data on health and medical care expenditures in the United States in the years 1929 and 1963. The estimated increase in expenditures of $30.2 billion is distributed among price, population, and "all other" (the last term incorporating changes in per capita use of services and in quality).

PERCENTAGE DISTRIBUTION AMONG FACTORS OF INCREASE IN
EXPENDITURES FOR HEALTH AND MEDICAL CARE IN THE
UNITED STATES, 1929–1963

Factor	Index Number		Annual Rate
	Method 1 (1)	Method 3 (2)	Method 1 (3)
Price	37	62	38
Population	16	18	19
All other	47	20	43

Source: Herbert E. Klarman, "Financing Health and Medical Care," in Duncan Clark and Brian MacMahon, eds., Textbook on Preventive Medicine (ms), Table 2 and p. 60 (to be published by Little, Brown and Co., Boston, in 1965).

The results differ markedly. Columns 1 and 3 both show the contribution of price to be of the order of three eighths rather than approximately two thirds (Column 2), which is the ratio frequently reported [42, p. 168; 70]. The factor "all other" is shown to be relatively less important in Column 3 than in Column 1 because the virtual elimination of the interaction term serves to enhance the contribution of the smallest term, population.

There is no logical basis for according priority to price in the allocation procedure. If the factor "all other" received first priority, the results in Column 2 would be reversed, as follows:

	Percent
Price	15
Population	15
All other	70

The writer has recommended adoption of the following procedure for allocating an increase in expenditures among two or more factors, including price:

1. Employ index numbers.

2. Convert all figures into annual rates of change, thereby minimizing the interaction term. (Subtract 100 from the index number, to obtain the percentage change over the entire interval. Then convert this figure into an average annual rate of increase.)

3. Treat all factors simultaneously; that is, do not assign priority to any factor.

This procedure is obviously reproducible. It offers the further advantage of permitting the introduction of additional factors at any stage of the analysis, without affecting the computations already completed. Thus, the factor "all other" may be subdivided, to allow for improvement in quality or to take separate account of the above average use of health and medical services by aged persons (65 and over) [76, pp. 10–11].

Adjusting for Improvement in Quality

An underlying concept of the Consumer Price Index is that price changes are measured for goods and services of constant or equivalent quality. Thus, the Bureau of Labor Statistics makes a downward adjustment in the hospitalization insurance premium for that part of the increase that represents an expansion of benefits [207, p. 1,176]. For much of surgery pre- and postoperative care have come to be incorporated in the physician's bill. If so, an increase in quoted charges may not represent an increase in price but rather a change in product [216, p. 3].

Because so many new drugs and varieties of drugs are being steadily introduced, a new sample of drugs was selected in 1960 and substituted for the old one [207, p. 1182]. In 1961 obstetricians' fees for obstetrical care were substituted for those of general practitioners [225, p. 132]. The procedure by which drug prices and obstetricians' fees were adjusted for quality change is called linking. This consists of tying a price measure based on the new quality to the preceding one by factoring out the difference in price when both varieties of a product are available on the market at the same time [207, p. 1178]. Linking has been criticized as particularly inappropriate for medical care prices, since the consumer has little scope to implement a judgment as to which variety of a good or service he will buy [225, p. 133]. Arrow has observed that any rule that will adjust for quality changes in a price index must involve the exercise of judgment somewhere in the procedure and cannot be completely objective [190, p. 85].

Most economists who have dealt with medical care prices recognize the need to make an allowance for quality improvement [225, p. 131]. However, one economist experienced in measuring national income and prices objects to adjusting for improvement in quality, unless the use of scarce economic resources is involved. When scarce resources are not employed, a costless gain accrues that should not enter into economic calculations [203, p. 993]. Moreover, some improvements in quality, such as the shorter stay in hospitals due to early ambulation, represent corrections of prior mistakes in medical practice. Other students take the position that most improvements in mortality and morbidity reflect advances in the standard of living and in public health and are not attributable to medical care [212, pp. 75–76]. If so, there is little or no reason to adjust medical care prices for changes in quality.

The prevailing view seems to be that an allowance for quality improvement is in order. To do this the economist is peculiarly dependent on the physician and the nurse for guidance. In recent years a great deal has been written on the quality of medical care, but there is still no agreement on how to measure it [174, pp. 300–8]. Most appraisals of quality are based on the conditions surrounding the provision of care, such as the qualifications of staff, suitability of physical plant, accreditation, and so forth. For the most part it is not yet feasible to appraise quality on the basis of the end results, that is, the health of patients. A panel of consultants to the Veterans Administration found that an evaluation of medical care through the study of medical records is more concerned with improving care than with measuring quality [227, p. 2].

It is not evident what the economist should employ as an indicator of change in quality. Most commonly cited as a possible criterion is a change in the average duration of patient stay in the hospital [216, p. 5; 225, p. 139]. Fifteen years ago the British Working Party on Nurses was urged by a minority of its members to adopt a short stay as the criterion of effective performances by nurses. The Commission refused, on the ground that speedy discharge is not the same as effective treatment. In this country the average duration of patient stay in hospitals is shortest in the southeastern region and longest in the Middle Atlantic states. Is one to infer that the former states have the superior quality of care? Similarly in New York City the average duration of patient stay is appreciably longer in voluntary hospitals than in proprietary hospitals for the same diagnostic condition [146, pp. 233–34] and still longer in government hospitals. Is the ranking of hospital ownership groups according to duration of stay the same as their ranking according to what is known or believed about quality of care?

A good part of the reduction in average duration of stay, as distinguished from a shift in composition toward a higher proportion of short-stay patients, does not entail the use of scarce resources. To the extent that it does, however, it should be allowed for.

The writer attempted to calculate the additional cost of the heightened daily activity in the hospital that is associated with a shorter stay. For the period 1934–57 in New York City this factor was estimated at 7 percent of the unit cost increase [132, p. 229]; the figure may be on the low side, since only ancillary services were taken into account. Other estimates are much higher—of the order of 25 percent—but they are based on an arbitrary allocation of the increase in hospital expenditures among increases in quality, price, and use [193, p. 53].

B. COSTS AND BENEFITS OF HEALTH PROGRAMS

Health and medical services may represent an investment in human capital or final consumption [204, p. 283]. (One economist has suggested that health and medical care expenditures should be viewed as neither investment nor consumption, but as repair or maintenance expenditures on the human machine [14, p. 29]. The writer cannot agree: man is not a machine; and why should not other expenditures, including food, be treated similarly?)

The distinction between consumption and investment has serious implications for policy. If health and medical services are consumer goods, the best way to go about getting more of them is, first, to invest in those things that raise the national output and, then, to devote part of the increment to buying additional health services [213, p. 40]. Conversely, if health services are investment goods, it may be practicable to buy more of them directly.

Investment versus Consumption

Calculating the difference between economic benefits and costs is an obvious step in justifying expenditures on health and medical services as a form of investment [24, p. 785]. In the past this type of calculation was usually performed by public health officials [24, p. 788]. In recent years economists working on problems of health and medical care have come to regard the estimate of net economic yield as a guide to society's demand for health services [206, p. 1; 229, p. 28]. Many economists share the view that health and medical care expenditures are primarily an investment in human beings [51, p. 140; 200, p. 129; 205, p. 15]. Pigou has stated, "The most important investment of all is investment in the health, intelligence and character of the people" [28, p. 138].

Expenditures for medical care to diagnose and treat a disease (or injury) are not its total costs. The costs of a disease comprise at least two components: direct costs and indirect costs. Direct costs are the medical care expenditures associated with a disease. Indirect costs are the loss of output, attributable to the disease, that result from premature death or disability. (Some economists list additional losses, such as those due to debility [219, p. 801] and avoidance costs [229, p. 45]. However, these have not been measured.) It is possible to reduce direct costs by failing to provide services, but indirect costs continue [200, p. 128].

The total costs of a disease per case serve as the measure of benefits derived from preventing that case [229, p. 90]. In a cost-benefit calculation the comparison is between contemplated additional expenditures for health and medical services, on the one hand, and the anticipated reduction in costs (direct plus indirect), on the other hand. This is the essential conceptual framework. (Although Fein states in his study of mental illness that the focus is on costs [200, pp. 3, 5] and Weisbrod states in his study of cancer, poliomyelitis, and tuberculosis that it is limited to benefits [229, p. 5], both deal with the same problem in similar fashion.) In practice, difficulties may arise as decisions are made on the methods of handling the several elements of the calculation and, as compromises are struck, by measuring the elements for which data are available rather than those which are indicated by the conceptual framework or theoretical model.

Some economists view medical services, if not public health services, primarily as consumer goods [13, p. 119; 19, p. 29; 111, p. 32]. (Denison states that the great majority of employed persons in this country have access to reasonable medical care, so that there is not much prevailing illness that can be cured [6, p. 52]. The writer is more inclined to agree with the conclusion than with the premise.) The calculation is then reduced to a comparison of expenditures for alternative programs that promise the same degree of health improvement [3, p. 251; 220, p. 215].

One difficulty is that few (if any) health services are pure investment goods or pure consumption goods. It is customary to recognize the consumption benefit of most health and medical care expenditures, to comment on the difficulty of measuring it, and then to dismiss it [221, p. 393; 229, p. 29]. What is measurable may not be necessarily important, but it is recorded and, therefore, cited. The measurable part (the investment component) is not likely, however, to bear a uniform relationship to the consumption component in all health and medical care programs. Attaching a value to the consumption part of the benefit, lest it be totally neglected (or treated as zero), is a challenging task [218, p. 156].

A possible approach is through the device of the analogous disease (one that may be regarded as inflicting equal pain or discomfort [230, p. 139]). Consider a disease, B, for which medical care expenditures are incurred without any prospect of a return in increased output, either because the disease is not disabling or because the patient has retired from the labor force. These expenditures are incurred for consumption purposes only and may be held to indicate the value of the consumption benefit attached to avoiding or curing the disease A that is under study [209, p. 5].

In comparing programs for which both costs and benefits are pertinent, the ratio of benefits to costs is not the proper criterion for choosing among them. This is true in part because a ratio of benefits to costs in excess of one is an insufficient criterion for justifying a program, since other programs may show a higher ratio. The principal reason is that a ratio of annual gross receipts (benefits) to annual expenses is not the correct criterion for evaluation [215, p. 110]. The proper test is that the return on investment or, more precisely, the present worth of the project be maximized [215, p. 76]. (This is also the ultimate criterion for optimum behavior in business when the rate of profit fluctuates through time [43b, p. 150].)

The Rate of Discount

To repeat, the calculation of costs and benefits properly compares the present value of proposed costs and of expected benefits. If the time span is longer than one year, the two streams should be discounted to the present by means of an appropriate rate of interest. A given amount of money has different values when it is realized (or spent) at different times. Discounting converts a stream of costs or benefits into its present worth. The higher the rate of interest adopted for discounting, the lower the present value of a given money stream.

Discounting assumes particular importance when the time span is long. Waterworks are a good example of long-lived investments. Another is a syphilis control program, the benefits (prevention of disability and premature death) of which accrue 15 to 30 years after the costs are incurred [209, p. 6].

At what level should the rate of discount be set? Some economists employ the going market rate of interest [200, p. 73; 215, p. 79; 221, p. 398]. It is not clear whether this is always the appropriate rate. In general, the discount rate balances the productivity of an investment and time preference (reluctance to sacrifice current for future consumption) [208, p. 11]. But the sum of individual preferences in the market and the collective estimate of time preference need not agree. It may be necessary to employ a rate that synthesizes the social rate of discount and opportunity cost (investment foregone) in the private sector [201, p. 130; 208, p. 23]. Much work remains to be done in this area.

Pure time preference is likely to vary with the life expectancy of a population [199, p. 457]; it may also vary by socioeconomic class. An individual's discount rate for the distant future is likely to be higher than that of society [58, pp. 91–92], which has the greater regard for later generations.

Some economists see the selection of a discount rate as expressing a judgment on the relative importance of successive generations. Accordingly, they prefer to offer two alternatives— 4 percent and 10 percent [206, p. 6; 229, p. 57] or 4 percent and 8 percent [195, Chap. 5, p. 23].

In the writer's opinion, presenting two or more rates is justified when it is accompanied by criteria for selecting one of them as the appropriate rate under specified circumstances. In the absence of such criteria a single rate is preferable. The rate of 4 (or 6) percent has the advantages of being intermediate along the range of available figures, of wide application

[194, p. 76; 200, p. 87; 208, p. 11; 221, p. 398], and of immunity from obvious objections.

Calculating Health and Medical Care Expenditures for a Disease

The calculation of health and medical care expenditures associated with a disease presents fewer conceptual problems than the calculation of output loss attributable to a disease. The statistical task, may, however, be just as formidable.

One requirement is that the total costs of a program be entered, including the value of services rendered by capital in the current period.

It is necessary to deal with the problem of determining the costs of health programs produced together. The arbitrary allocation of overhead in order to determine the average unit cost of several jointly produced services does not contribute to sound decisions [43a, pp. 306–7; 108, pp. 359–60; 215, pp. 44–45].

Data by disease classification are scarce, especially in private medical practice. Moreover, several diseases may be associated in a person at the same time. Yet, the summary page of the medical record of a hospitalized patient may report only his primary diagnosis (the final diagnosis of the condition for which the patient was admitted).

The presence of associated conditions (or multiple diseases) also poses a difficulty in estimating the contemplated effect of proposed expenditures on alternative programs of health services. Even if all multiple diseases were correctly reported, their simultaneous presence implies overstatement of the economic cost of any disease taken singly and, therefore, overstatement of the potential savings to be achieved by reducing the incidence of any one disease [216, p. 9; 219, p. 802].

Another, similar difficulty is presented by competing causes of death. This difficulty is manifested in the uncertainties that surround the preparation of a life table from which a given cause of death is removed [229, pp. 34–35]. Moreover, if the effect of a program is to prolong life expectancy, morbidity may also rise [206, p. 12].

Owing to the presence of multiple diseases and of competing causes of death, it is a mistake to add the calculated costs of individual diseases in an attempt to estimate the total cost of disease to a society [219, p. 802].

Calculating Output Loss

The calculation of the indirect costs of a disease or injury presents several problems. Among them are the treatment of transfer payments, taxes, consumption, the work of housewives, the appropriate measure of output loss, and the choice of assumptions regarding employment as well as the discount rate. About some of these elements of cost students of the economic costs of road accidents, mental illness, cancer, tuberculosis, poliomyelitis, ulcers, alcoholism, and job accidents are approaching a consensus. Differences of opinion and in approach persist regarding others.

Transfer payments. The consensus revolves about the treatment of transfer payments, taxes, and the measure of output loss. When expenditures are incurred without any cost in resources, they constitute transfer payments. Since transfer payments do not entail a change in resource cost to the community, they represent a redistribution of income within the community and a shift in command over resources. Once resource loss is taken into account, there is no reason to bring transfer payments into the calculation [219, p. 801]. If relief checks are replaced by earnings as the source of family support, it is the earnings that measure society's gain in output. To count the reduction in relief grants as well is to count this amount twice. The social desirability of having families live on their own earnings, rather than on relief grants, does not enter into this calculation; it may be entitled to separate recognition.

Taxes. The argument concerning the proper treatment of taxes is similar. It is double counting to include tax receipts by government once earnings have been counted. Although some may disagree [195, p. 131], the amount of taxes and the distribution of the burden of taxes have no proper bearing on decisions made concerning health and medical care programs, unless the beneficiaries are subject to a special tax. It would perhaps be realistic to recognize that the proposed expenditures may fall on one pocketbook while the potential benefits accrue to other pocketbooks or are widely diffused [200, p. 132; 206, p. 4; 222, pp. 12–13].

Earnings. Increasingly regarded as the appropriate measure of output loss are the earnings of employed members of the labor force (wages and salaries and net income from self-employment) [192, p. 18; 200, p. 69; 229, p. 49]. To count total output per employed member of the labor force, as some economists do [221, p. 396], is tantamount to attributing to labor the entire output of the economy [219, p. 805].

Owing to continuing improvement in the economy's productivity, future earnings per worker are almost certain to exceed current earnings (in real terms, that is, apart from a rise in the general price level). If an average (geometric) annual rate of gain in productivity is projected, it can be conveniently applied as a partial offset to the discount rate [209, p. 13; 218, p. 148].

Rate of unemployment. A difference of opinion prevails regarding the rate of unemployment to assume for the beneficiaries of a health program. The current consensus favors the assumption of full employment (4 percent unemployment). The justification is that, if a health program is effective in preventing or curing a disease and makes people available for productive employment, then the program has achieved its objective [219, p. 801].

Yet it seems reasonable to suppose that even in a period of full employment there may be a difference in employment potential between a group of persons in whom a disease has been prevented and one in whom that disease occurs and is cured. Past job history may also be a factor.

The applicability of the full employment assumption to developing countries has been challenged. The economic benefit of preventing premature death depends on whether a survivor is in fact offered productive work [220, p. 211]. The economic value of health reform depends on the rate of economic development; it can be negative in a stagnant system [220, p. 214].

Consumption. Wide differences of opinion obtain regarding the treatment of consumption. Economists agree that in calculating the economic value of a man insurance companies should deduct his consumption [194, pp. 76–82]. Unlike insurance companies or the man's family, however, society as a whole is concerned with total output, of which consumption is a part [219, p. 806]. After all, it is consumption that is the end (goal) of economic activity [200, pp. 19–20]. According to this view, net earnings after consumption are irrelevant to the economist's central concern, and consumption should not be deducted from gross earnings in estimating the gain in output attributable to a health program.

It has been stated that the treatment of consumption depends on one's definition of society, that is, whether the potential survivor is regarded as a member. If he is, consumption should not be deducted from earnings; and conversely [229, pp. 35–36]. Weisbrod does not explicitly choose between the two definitions. However, he develops elaborate and carefully calculated estimates of consumption and employs them in the estimates of economic loss [229, p. 84].

Some economists deduct consumption as a matter of course, without explanation [210, p. 130; 221, p. 396]. In their work the calculation of benefits can result in a negative figure, such as Laitin's finding for cancer among the aged [210, p. 130]. This finding has been erroneously interpreted to mean that killing of the ill may be economically desirable—a repugnant notion [192, p. 18; 201, p. 129].

How to treat consumption is a problem because a health program affects not only a nation's output but also the size of population. It is necessary to distinguish between a program that saves people from death to perform useful labor and one that saves people from death to pursue an unproductive life.

In a poor nation it would seem important to pose a clear-cut choice between programs, in terms of their effect on per capita output. In this country it may not be necessary to pose such a choice. If it is, separate weights might be attached to changes in per capita output and in aggregate output. The relative magnitudes of these weights is a matter for political decision.

The above approach would lend consistency to the position of those economists who consider the deduction of consumption invalid for the United States but deem it necessary to deduct the minimum essential consumption of survivors in a developing country [219, p. 807].

The medical care expenditures in behalf of a survivor in an institution automatically include his ordinary expenditures as a consumer. These should be deducted to the extent that his family makes downward adjustments in its own expenditures [195, Chap. 2, p. 16]. Such adjustments are more likely to be associated with long-term institutional care than with short-term hospitalization.

Services of housewives. Differences of opinion prevail regarding the proper treatment of the services of housewives. Those who would disregard them acknowledge a serious understatement of the costs of some diseases but justify the exclusion on two grounds. It is difficult to measure the value of the services of housewives, since they occur outside the market mechanism. The imputation (attributing the equivalent of a market price where none exists) of economic value raises too many statistical problems [200, pp. 23–24, 143]. To include the services of housewives is also inconsistent with the accepted procedures of national income accounting [219, pp. 803–4].

Others prefer to include the economic contribution of housewives, despite the complexities involved [192, p. 18; 221, p. 396; 229, p. 56]. When the housewife is sick, it costs money to hire a replacement. The housewife's services must be counted in comparing costs among diseases, for the distribution of diseases between the sexes is not uniform. To disregard the services of housewives in calculating output loss is to understate the economic benefits of a health program that serves a preponderantly female population. Moreover, if the costs of several diseases are not additive, there is no occasion to relate the total costs of all diseases to the national output.

One economist measures the value of housewives' services in terms of the cost of a housekeeper replacement who would assume responsibility for running the same size of household [229, p. 70]. From a practical standpoint it is simpler to employ the earnings of a domestic servant. This amount is on the low side, but it offsets the tendency to overvalue a product not sold in the market when it is assigned the price of a counterpart [18, p. 22–23, 432].

Application of the Cost-Benefit Calculation

In his book Weisbrod develops estimates of costs for three diseases—cancer, poliomyelitis, and tuberculosis. For each disease he calculates separately the direct costs of medical care and the loss of net earnings due to premature death and sickness (disability). He then states the general rule for the optimum allocation of funds among disease programs, namely, that the ratios of marginal benefit (the benefit of preventing an additional case of a disease) to marginal cost (the cost of preventing an additional case) should be equal [229, p. 88]. This criterion is tantamount to requiring equal benefits to accrue from spending one additional dollar on each disease [229, p. 63].

It is not possible, however, to eliminate each of the three diseases. A given program in cancer is likely to have only a partial effect on morbidity. It is the benefit of the partial reduction in morbidity that should be measured [201, pp. 129–30], with due cognizance of the continuing costs, if any, of a surveillance program.

For the final calculation of cost and benefit it is necessary to have an estimate of the cost of preventing an additional case of disease. The cost of case finding may be high (both financially and psychologically) even when a highly sensitive test is available, if the prevalence rate of the disease is fairly low. For example, Wallis and Roberts assume an annual incidence of cancer of 5 per 1,000 population (not an unrealistic figure at the middle ages) and a test for detecting cancer that possesses a high degree of reliability, say 95 percent. Under these conditions only 1 in 11 or 12 persons with positive reactions to the test would really have the disease, and the others would be falsely identified as positive [50, pp. 328–29]. Screening tests yield a larger economic benefit to the community when the morbidity rate is higher [191, pp. 358–59].

In considering a new health program, expenditures of effort and money should be related to possible accomplishments. "Diseases of the circulatory system may be the most important cause of death in a community but these conditions are not affected by known preventive measures to the same extent as typhoid fever" [26, p. 232].

It goes without saying that economic arithmetic is only one factor in evaluating programs of health services. Ultimately the preservation of life and the alleviation of pain represent value judgments. It may be that the cost-benefit calculation is useful as an affirmative argument in support of a program and not so useful as an argument against a program that is advocated on humanitarian or other grounds. The question has been raised whether the investment criterion may not be taken as a minimum one, that is, as setting a floor to the size of a proposed health services program [204, p. 283; 221, p. 403; 229, p. 94].

Applications to Medical Research

It has been proposed that the allocation of research funds among diseases should be similar to the ranking of diseases by economic loss [200, p. 124; 229, p. 87]. This policy was recommended to the federal government shortly after World War II, as follows: "The (medical research) problems under investigation should bear a reasonably close relation to those questions of illness and death which are most common in the population" [217, p. 423].

It is questionable on several grounds whether research funds should be allocated among diseases in relation to the severity of the economic problems they present. This view neglects differences at a given time in the expected difficulty and cost of making comparable improvements in the prevention or treatment of different diseases [217, p. 424]. In evaluating a research proposal the appropriate question is whether, in the present state of knowledge and techniques, it offers a promising lead or chance of further development [201, p. 130]. Nor is it desirable to turn research efforts on and off at will, as the calculated criteria for the allocation of funds change [192, p. 58].

Also to be considered is the large contribution to health advances made by basic research. Ginzberg asserts flatly that most of the outstanding advances in health research have been by-products of basic research in biology, chemistry, physics, and the other sciences [12, p. 735]. Others have noted that basic research is the foundation upon which all other research rests [223, p. 154]; and the uncertainty of discovery is such that it is not possible to buy the specific discoveries one wants [15, p. 71].

Finally, a given health services program may receive dividends from many and unexpected directions. Consider the field of psychiatry. Mental diseases due to nutritional deficiency were eliminated when a vitamin was discovered as a cure and preventive for pellagra. Paresis (a wasting disease of the central nervous system caused by syphilis) is being eliminated by penicillin. The tranquilizing drugs derive from research in diseases of the circulatory system.

The limiting factor in medical research today is not money but scientists [6, p. 53; 13, p. 113; 212, p. 174]. Some believe that there are not enough qualified men available to carry out the work that Congress wishes to pay for with the appropriations it votes [223, p. 156], so that research in one field is performed at the cost of neglecting another. Support and expansion of training [6, p. 52; 15, p. 71; 192, p. 58] are, therefore, prerequisite— both logically and in time—to the effective expansion of research. (Some grounds for government spending on research are noted in Chapter III, Section B.)

C. WHAT CAN WE AFFORD TO SPEND?

There are those who regard human life as beyond economic calculation and would not stint in spending money on health and medical care. This position was well expressed some years ago by a Blue Cross executive. No amount of money paid to doctors and hospitals is enough, because they are "engaged in the Lord's work, and they see no end to the things that should be done for suffering humanity" [228, p. 407].

Today an open-ended attitude toward health and medical care expenditures is likely to take the form of urging additional investment in health services. Health is purchasable, it is argued, and it is a good buy. The larger the expenditure, the more health there will be. The expenditure is said to be self-liquidating in that it increases the productivity of the labor force and, hence, the national income [51, p. 140; 200, p. 129]. There are economists, however, who believe that few health and medical expenditures in this country partake of the nature of an investment and that most such expenditures represent consumption [6, pp. 51–52; 13, p. 119; 19, p. 29; 111, p. 32].

People have many wants, and it is incumbent on every society to economize in the use of scarce resources. Economists agree that a nation can always afford to spend more on (devote more resources to) health and medical care, provided it is willing to spend less on other things [13, p. 115; 60, p. 285; 200, p. 137; 229, p. vii]. (Note the implicit assumption of "full" employment.) Nevertheless, no nation, however affluent, can afford to apply all the known scientific measures for relieving pain, preventing or curing illness, and postponing death. To at least one economist it is inconceivable that any society will ever be rich enough to eliminate all the eliminable (postponable) causes of death [43b, p. 2].

It has been said that in this country consumers display their preferences in the market when they choose to spend only four percent of disposable income on medical care and many billions of dollars on such items as liquor and tobacco [198, p. 18]. The implication is that, if the American public wanted more health and medical services, it would spend more money on them and less on other things.

Several comments are in order. There is no evidence that medical care and liquor and tobacco are close competitors in a family's budget at a given time. Bills for medical care occur irregularly and are highly concentrated, while expenditures for liquor and tobacco are regular and small. Furthermore, consumer expenditures for liquor and tobacco are in part joint products with health and medical care expenditures by government, since tax revenues from the former help to pay for the latter [205, p. 13]. Finally, consumers no longer spend 4 percent of their income on health and medical care but closer to 6 percent [31, p. 6].

This nation is spending a great deal more money on health and medical care today than formerly. It is spending more than some of the published figures indicate or than many of us realize, both in absolute amount and in relation to the national product. As expenditures for health and medical care increase, it is necessary to face two questions. Is the additional money eliciting a commensurate flow of services or merely serving to raise prices? If additional services are elicited, do they improve the health of the population? The first question lies more in the realm of economics than the second. But even the second question has certain economic aspects, since it calls for comparisons with the costs of other programs, such as nutrition or education, that may be deemed capable of yielding the same degree of health improvement. Such a comparison would perhaps spotlight the gap between our aspiration for better health and the ability of modern medicine to deliver it [12, p. 742]. Of course, a wealthy nation can afford to spend more to eliminate discomfort and pain than a poor nation and may choose to do so [19, p. 38].

Ultimately the decision on how much to spend on health and medical services as consumption goods is one of value judgment. Investment aspects apart, there are no economic criteria for choosing between more medical care and more schools, housing, recreation, and so forth [3, pp. 250–51].

In this country the decision is multiple, involving many buyers in every sector of the economy. The behavior of the buyers is influenced by their financial means—income in the case of consumers, tax inducements and collective bargaining arrangements in the case of business, and tax revenues and borrowing power in the case of government. Another determinant of expenditures is the opportunity (or lack of one) to prepay periodically in small amounts for an adequate range of benefits. Prepayment facilitates spending and expands the base from which expenditures are made. Not only does the consumer designate a given sum for this purpose when he is well and pays the health insurance premium, but the sense of security afforded by the prospect of insurance benefits apparently influences him to spend more on those health and medical services that are not insured. Prepayment also broadens the base of financing by permitting employer participation in the premium.

The fact that funds for health and medical care derive from many pocketbooks is of prime importance. To deal with finances in the aggregate, as if all monies came from one pocketbook and were under a single control, is to indulge in a gross oversimplification. At a given time some sources of funds have greater access to additional monies than others. Occasionally the several sources may compete with one another for achievement and status.

Economists have observed that in the real world the issue is seldom, if ever, the total amount that a nation or group might spend for a given purpose, but whether it should spend more or less than currently. They start with what is and proceed to consider alternatives step by step, by small increment or decrement. Not only is this approach sound for the economist; it is also constructive politically, since it permits adjustments and compromises [3, p. 55].

Even step by step decisions are not made simply. A society's goals are many and sometimes conflicting. Our society cannot be said to be single-minded in the pursuit of health. The public's demand for high quality health and medical services may outrun its willingness to devote a sufficiently large portion of the national output to this purpose [34, p. 403]. Perhaps more important, at a given time and place the roads to health are many, and increased expenditures for health and medical care are only one of them. Finally, there are certain items of consumption, such as food or recreation, that are in themselves desirable or pleasurable and also contribute to better health. There are other items of consumption, such as a stay in the hospital or nursing home, that are not desired for themselves and would not be purchased if they were not essential. The writer believes that, in general, a balanced pattern of expenditures is likely to make a greater contribution to a people's health than emphasis on some single object of expenditures.

SELECTED BIBLIOGRAPHY

A. GENERAL

1. Kenneth E. Boulding. *Principles of Economic Policy.* Englewood Cliffs, N. J., Prentice Hall, 1958.
2. James M. Buchanan. *The Public Finances.* Homewood, Ill., Richard Irwin, 1960.
3. Jesse Burkhead. *Government Budgeting.* New York, John Wiley, 1956.
4. Council of Economic Advisers. *Annual Report, 1962.* Washington, D.C., Government Printing Office, 1962.
5. Michael M. Davis. *Medical Care for Tomorrow.* New York, Harper, 1955.
6. Edward F. Denison. *The Sources of Economic Growth in the United States and the Alternatives before Us.* Supplementary Paper No. 13 by Committee for Economic Development. New York, 1962.
7. J. Frederic Dewhurst and Associates. *America's Needs and Resources.* New York, The Twentieth Century Fund.
   a. 1947.
   b. *A New Survey*, 1955.
8. Rene Dubos. *Mirage of Health.* New York, Harper, 1959.
9. *The Economist.* American Survey, "Bill of Health," 4 Parts, August 29, September 19, October 10, and October 24, 1959.
10. Martin S. Feldstein. "Economic Analysis, Operational Research, and the National Health Service," *Oxford Economic Papers*, 14: No. 1 (March, 1963), 19–31.
11. Milton Friedman. *Price Theory: A Provisional Text.* Chicago, Aldine, 1962.
12. Eli Ginzberg. "Health, Medicine, and Economic Welfare," *Journal of the Mount Sinai Hospital*, 19: No. 6 (March-April, 1953), 734–43.
13. Eli Ginzberg. "What Every Economist Should Know About Health and Medicine," *American Economic Review*, 44: No. 1 (March, 1954), 104–19.
14. Harry I. Greenfield. *Medical Care in the United States: an Economic Work-up.* Paper delivered at annual meeting of the American Association for the Advancement of Science, Cleveland, Ohio, December 26, 1963.

15. Alan Gregg. *Challenges to Contemporary Medicine*. New York, Columbia University Press, 1956.

16. Alvin H. Hansen. "Trends and Cycles in Economic Activity." *Review of Economics and Statistics*, 39: No. 2 (May, 1957), 105–15.

17. John Jewkes and Sylvia Jewkes. *The Genesis of the British National Health Service*. Oxford, Blackwell, 1961.

18. Simon Kuznets. *National Income and Its Composition, 1919–1938*. New York, National Bureau of Economic Research, 1947.

19. D. S. Lees. *Health through Choice*. London, Institute of Economic Affairs, 1961.

20. Thomas McKeown and R. G. Brown. "Medical Evidence Related to English Population Changes in the Eighteenth Century," *Population Studies*, 9: No. 2 (November, 1955), 119–41.

21. Ida C. Merriam. "Social Welfare Expenditures, 1960–1961," *Social Security Bulletin*, 25: No. 11 (November, 1962), 3–13.

22. Charlotte Muller. "Economic Analysis of Medical Care in the United States," *American Journal of Public Health*, 51: No. 1 (January, 1961), 31–42.

23. Richard A. Musgrave. *The Theory of Public Finance*. New York, McGraw Hill, 1959.

24. Selma J. Mushkin. "Toward a Definition of Health Economics," *Public Health Reports*, 73: No. 9 (September, 1958), 785–93.

25. Selma J. Mushkin. "Why Health Economics?" in *The Economics of Health and Medical Care*. Ann Arbor, Mich., Bureau of Public Health Economics and Department of Economics, The University of Michigan, 1964. Pp. 3–13.

26. Thomas Parran, Harry S. Mustard, Dean A. Clark, eds., *Selected Papers of Joseph W. Mountin*. Washington, D.C., Joseph W. Mountin Memorial Committee, 1956.

27. A. C. Pigou. *Economics in Practice*. London, Macmillan, 1935.

28. A. C. Pigou. *Socialism vs. Capitalism*. London, Macmillan, 1947.

29. President's Commission on the Health Needs of the Nation. *Building America's Health*. Vols. 1–5. Washington, D.C., Superintendent of Documents, 1952.

30. Herbert Ratner. *Medicine, Interview on the American Character*. Santa Barbara, Calif., Center for the Study of Democratic Institutions, 1962.

31. Louis S. Reed and Dorothy P. Rice. "Private Medical Care Expenditures and Voluntary Health Insurance, 1948–61," *Social Security Bulletin*, 25: No. 12 (December, 1962), 3–13.

32. Ffrangcon Roberts. *The Cost of Health*. London, Turnstile Press, 1952.

33. Joan Robinson. *The Economics of Imperfect Competition.* London, Macmillan, 1946.
34. Earl R. Rolph and George F. Break. *Public Finance.* New York, Ronald Press, 1961.
35. Jerome Rothenberg. *The Measurement of Social Welfare.* Englewood Cliffs, N. J., Prentice Hall, 1961.
36. Paul A. Samuelson. *Economics.* New York, McGraw Hill.
    a. First edition, 1948.
    b. Third edition, 1955.
    c. Fifth edition, 1961.
37. Tibor Scitovsky. *Welfare and Competition.* Chicago, Richard Irwin, 1951.
38. J. R. Seale. "A General Theory of National Expenditure on Medical Care," *The Lancet,* No. 7, 102 (October 10, 1959), 555–59.
39. William J. Shultz and C. Lowell Harriss. *American Public Finance.* 7th ed., Englewood Cliffs, N. J., Prentice Hall, 1959.
40. Adam Smith. *The Wealth of Nations.* New York, Random House, 1937.
41. Arthur Smithies. "Federal Budgeting and Fiscal Policy," in Howard S. Ellis, ed., *A Survey of Contemporary Economics.* Philadelphia, Blakiston, 1948. Pp. 174–209.
42. Herman Miles Somers and Anne Ramsay Somers. *Doctors, Patients and Health Insurance.* Washington, D.C., The Brookings Institution, 1961.
43. George J. Stigler. *The Theory of Price.* New York, Macmillan.
    a. First edition, 1946.
    b. Revised edition, 1952.
44. George J. Stigler. *Trends in Employment in the Service Industries.* Princeton, N. J., Princeton University Press, 1956.
45. U. S. National Health Survey. *Health Statistics, Veterans, Health and Medical Care, United States, July, 1957–June, 1958,* Series C – No. 2. Washington, D.C., Government Printing Office, 1960.
46. U. S. Public Health Service. *Health Manpower Source Book, Section 7, Dentists.* Washington, D.C., Government Printing Office, 1955.
47. U. S. Public Health Service, Division of Public Health Methods, *Chart Book on Health Status and Health Manpower.* Washington, D.C., Government Printing Office, 1961.
48. U. S. Public Health Service. Division of Hospital and Medical Facilities. Press Release, November 9, 1962.
49. U. S. Public Health Service. Press Release on Physician-Population Ratios, September 6, 1963.

50. W. Allen Wallis and Harry V. Roberts. *Statistics: A New Approach.* Glencoe, Ill., The Free Press, 1956.
51. Burton A. Weisbrod. "Anticipating the Health Needs of Americans: Some Economic Projections," *Annals of the American Academy of Political and Social Science,* 337 (September, 1961), 137–45.

B. DEMAND AND FINANCING

52. Brian Abel-Smith and R. M. Titmuss. *The Cost of the National Health Service in England and Wales.* Cambridge, England, Cambridge University Press, 1956.
53. Odin W. Anderson, Patricia Collette, and Jacob J. Feldman. *Changes in Family Medical Care Expenditures and Voluntary Health Insurance.* Cambridge, Mass., Harvard University Press, 1963.
54. Odin W. Anderson and Jacob J. Feldman. *Family Medical Costs and Voluntary Health Insurance: A Nationwide Survey.* New York, McGraw Hill, 1956.
55. Kenneth J. Arrow. "Uncertainty and the Welfare Economics of Medical Care," *American Economic Review,* 53: No. 5 (December, 1963), 941–73.
56. Francis M. Bator. *The Question of Government Spending.* New York, Collier Books, 1960.
57. Peter T. Bauer and Basil S. Yamey. *The Economics of Underdeveloped Countries.* Chicago, University of Chicago Press, 1957.
58. William J. Baumol. *Welfare Economics and the Theory of the State.* Cambridge, Mass., Harvard University Press, 1952.
59. Benjamin J. Darsky, Nathan Sinai, and Solomon J. Axelrod. *Comprehensive Medical Services under Voluntary Health Insurance.* Cambridge, Mass., Harvard University Press, 1958.
60. James S. Duesenberry. "Government Expenditures and Growth," in *Federal Expenditure Policy for Economic Growth and Stability,* Joint Economic Committee, 85th Congress, 1st session, 1957. Pp. 285–91.
61. I. S. Falk, C. Rufus Rorem, and Martha D. Ring. *The Costs of Medical Care.* Chicago, University of Chicago Press, 1933.
62. Paul J. Feldstein and Ruth M. Severson. "The Demand for Medical Care," in *Report of the Commission on the Cost of Medical Care,* Vol. I. Chicago, American Medical Association, 1964. Pp. 57–76.
63. Joseph W. Garbarino. *Health Plans and Collective Bargaining,* Berkeley, Calif., University of California Press, 1960.

64. Eli Ginzberg. "Federal Hospitalization," reprinted from *Modern Hospital*, 1949.
   a. Vol. 72, No. 4 (April), pp. 61–64.
   b. Vol. 73, No. 2 (August), pp. 73–74, 124–30.
   c. Vol. 73, No. 6 (December), pp. 43–47.
65. Harold M. Groves. "Economic and Public Finance Aspects of the Medical Care Problem," in *Financing a Health Program for America*, Vol. 4 of President's Commission on Health Needs of the Nation, *Building America's Health*. Washington, D.C., Superintendent of Documents, 1952. Pp. 142–46.
66. Robert Hamlin (Study Director). *Voluntary Health and Welfare Agencies in the United States*, An Exploratory Study by an Ad Hoc Citizens Committee. New York, The Schoolmasters Press, 1961.
67. Seymour E. Harris. *The Economics of American Medicine*. New York, Macmillan, 1964.
68. Seymour E. Harris. "Medical Care Expenditures in Relation to Family Income and National Income," in *Financing a Health Program for America*, Vol. 4 of President's Commission on the Health Needs of the Nation, *Building America's Health*. Washington, D.C., Superintendent of Documents, 1952. Pp. 3–16.
69. Charles G. Hayden, "An Evaluation of Blue Shield Plans," in *Financing a Health Program for America*, Vol. 4 of President's Commission on the Health Needs of the Nation, *Building America's Health*. Washington, D.C., Superintendent of Documents, 1952. Pp. 47–54.
70. Health Information Foundation. "Financing Further Progress," *Progress in Health Services*, 12: No. 1 (January-February, 1963).
71. Helen Hollingsworth, Margaret C. Klem, and Anna Mae Baney. *Medical Care Costs in Relation to Family Income*. Washington, D.C., Social Security Administration, Federal Security Agency, 1947.
72. C. Harry Kahn. "Personal Deductions in the Individual Income Tax," *Tax Revision Compendium*, Vol. 1, House Ways and Means Committee, November, 1959. Pp. 391–406.
73. C. Harry Kahn. *Personal Deductions in the Federal Income Tax*. Princeton, N. J., Princeton University Press, 1960.
74. Reuben A. Kessel, "Price Discrimination in Medicine," *Journal of Law and Economics,* 1 (October, 1958), 20–53.
75. a. Herbert E. Klarman. *Changing Costs of Medical Care and Voluntary Health Insurance*. Extended version of paper delivered before joint session of American Economic Association and American Association of University Teachers of Insurance, Cleveland, Ohio, December 28, 1956.

b. Herbert E. Klarman, "Medical Care Costs and Voluntary Health Insurance," *Journal of Insurance*, 24: No. 1 (September, 1957), 23–41.

76. Herbert E. Klarman. "Financing Health and Medical Care," in Duncan Clark and Brian MacMahon, eds., *Textbook on Preventive Medicine*. Boston, Little, Brown, 1965 (manuscript).

77. Clarence A. Kulp. "Voluntary and Compulsory Medical Care Insurance," *American Economic Review, Papers and Proceedings*, 41: No. 2 (May, 1951), 667–75.

78. Robert J. Lampman and S. F. Miyamoto. "Effects of Coverage of Home and Office Calls in a Physician-Sponsored Health Insurance Plan," *Journal of Insurance*, 28: No. 3 (September, 1961), 1–16.

79. Monroe Lerner. "Mortality and Morbidity in the United States as Basic Indices of Health Needs," *Annals of the American Academy of Political and Social Science*, 337 (September, 1961), 1–10.

80. Duncan M. MacIntyre. *Voluntary Health Insurance and Rate Making*. Ithaca, N. Y., Cornell University Press, 1962.

81. Julius Margolis, "A Comment on the Pure Theory of Public Expenditures," *Review of Economics and Statistics*, 37: No. 4 (November, 1955), 347–49.

82. Louis J. Paradiso and Clement Winston. "Consumer Expenditure-Income Patterns," *Survey of Current Business*, 35: No. 9 (September, 1955), 23–32.

83. Joseph A. Pechman. "The Individual Income Tax Base," in *Proceedings of the Forty-Eighth Annual Conference of the National Tax Association*. Sacramento, Calif., 1956. Pp. 304–15.

84. Louis S. Reed. *Medical Care under the New York Workmen's Compensation Program*. Ithaca, N. Y., Sloan Institute of Hospital Administration, Graduate School of Business and Public Administration, Cornell University, 1960.

85. Margaret G. Reid. *Housing and Income*. Chicago, University of Chicago Press, 1962.

86. Gaston V. Rimlinger, "Health Care of the Aged: Who Pays the Bill?" *Harvard Business Review*, 38: No. 1 (January-February, 1960), 108–16.

87. Alice M. Rivlin. *The Role of the Federal Government in Financing Higher Education*. Washington, D.C., The Brookings Institution, 1961.

88. Robert L. Robertson, Jr. National Aggregate Statistics on Expenditures for Medical Care. M.S. thesis, University of Wisconsin, Madison, Wis., 1956.

89. Robert L. Robertson, Jr. "The Market for Hospital Care," *Hospital Administration*, 7: No. 1 (Winter, 1962), 41–55.

90. Milton I. Roemer and Max Shain. *Hospital Utilization under Insurance.* Chicago, American Hospital Association, 1959.

91. C. Rufus Rorem. "Nonprofit Hospital Service Plans," *Medical Care,* 1: No. 2 (April, 1941), 135–47.

92. Jerome Rothenberg. "Welfare Implications of Alternative Methods of Financing Medical Care," *American Economic Review, Papers and Proceedings,* 41: No. 2 (May, 1951), 676–87.

93. Howard A. Rusk and Eugene J. Taylor. "Rehabilitation," *Annals of the American Academy of Political and Social Science,* 273 (January, 1951), 138–43.

94. Paul A. Samuelson. "The Pure Theory of Public Expenditure," *Review of Economics and Statistics,* 36: No. 4 (November, 1954), 387–89.

95. Herman Miles Somers and Anne Ramsay Somers. *Workmen's Compensation.* New York, John Wiley, 1954.

96. Malcolm G. Taylor. *Health Insurance in Canada.* Toronto, Oxford University Press, 1956.

97. U. S. Social Security Administration, Division of Program Research. *The Health Care of the Aged.* Washington, D.C., Government Printing Office, 1962.

98. U. S. Veterans Administration and Bureau of the Budget. *Current and Projected Veteran Patient Load through 1986.* Washington, D.C., The Bureau, 1958.

99. William S. Vickrey. "Resource Distribution Patterns and the Classification of Families," in *Studies in Income and Wealth,* Vol. 10. New York, National Bureau of Economic Research, 1947. Pp. 266–96.

100. William S. Vickrey. "One Economist's View of Philanthropy," in Frank G. Dickinson, ed., *Philanthropy and Public Policy.* New York, National Bureau of Economic Research, 1962. Pp. 31–56.

101. Burton A. Weisbrod and Robert J. Fiesler. "Hospitalization Insurance and Hospital Utilization," *American Economic Review,* 51: No. 1 (March, 1961), 126–32.

102. Melvin I. White. "Proper Income Tax Treatment of Deduction for Personal Expense," *Tax Revision Compendium,* Vol. 1, House Ways and Means Committee, November, 1959. Pp. 365–74.

103. Abba S. Yousri. Prepayment of Medical and Surgical Care Costs in Wisconsin. Ph.D. Dissertation, University of Wisconsin, Madison, Wis., 1956.

C. MANPOWER AND FACILITIES

104. Ralph E. Adams. *A Market Study of Hospital House Officers.* Chicago, Graduate Program in Hospital Administration, University of Chicago, 1961.

105. American Hospital Association. *Hospitals*, Guide Issue, 36: No. 15 (August 1, 1962).

106. Anonymous. "The Income of Physicians: A Comparison of Published Studies," *Medical Care*, 4: No. 3 (August, 1944), 221–27.

107. Frank Bane (for the Surgeon General's Consultant Group on Medical Education). *Physicians for a Growing America*. Washington, D.C., Government Printing Office, 1959.

108. William J. Baumol, and others. "The Role of Cost in the Minimum Pricing of Railroad Services," *Journal of Business*, 35: No. 4 (October, 1962), 357–66.

109. Mark Berke. "No Defense Needed," *Hospitals*, 32: No. 16 (August 16, 1958), 37.

110. David S. Blank and George J. Stigler. *The Demand and Supply of Scientific Personnel*. New York, National Bureau of Economic Research, 1957.

111. Kenneth E. Boulding. "An Economist's View of the Manpower Concept," in National Manpower Council, *Proceedings of a Conference on the Utilization of Scientific and Professional Manpower*. New York, Columbia University Press, 1954. Pp. 11–26.

112. Ray E. Brown. "The Nature of Hospital Costs," *Hospitals*, 30: No. 7 (April 1, 1956), 36–41.

113. Ray E. Brown. "A Current Evaluation of Hospital Planning," in U. S. Public Health Service, *Principles for Planning the Future Hospital System*. Washington, D.C., Government Printing Office, 1959. Pp. 23–31.

114. Antonio Ciocco, Burnet M. Davis, and Isidore Altman. "Measures of Medical Resources and Requirements," *Medical Care*, 3: No. 4 (November, 1943), 314–26.

115. Committee on the Function of Nursing. *A Program for the Nursing Profession*. New York, Macmillan, 1948.

116. William F. Damrau. The Rise of Municipal Hospital Expenditures in New York City, 1914–1954. Ph.D. Dissertation, New York University, New York, 1957.

117. Frank G. Dickinson. *Supply of Physicians' Services*. Bulletin 81. Chicago, Bureau of Medical Economic Research, American Medical Association, 1951.

118. Frank G. Dickinson. *How Bad is the Distribution of Physicians?* Bulletin 94B. Chicago, Bureau of Medical Economic Research, American Medical Association, 1954.

119. Marius Farioletti. "Some Income Adjustment Results from the 1949 Audit Control Program," in *An Appraisal of the 1950 Census Income Data*, Vol. 23, Studies in Income and Wealth. Princeton, N. J., Princeton University Press. Pp. 239–70.

120. Rashi Fein. Factors Influencing the Location of North Carolina General Medical Practitioners: A Study in Physician Distribution. Ph.D. Dissertation, Johns Hopkins University, Baltimore, Md., 1956.

121. Paul J. Feldstein. *An Empirical Investigation of the Marginal Cost of Hospital Services*. Chicago, Graduate Program in Hospital Administration, University of Chicago, 1961.

122. Gary L. Filerman. *A Comparative Study of the Utilization of Certain Hospital Services by Geriatric and Other Adult Patients, Staying Thirty Days or Less, in a General Acute Teaching Hospital*. Baltimore, Md., Operations Research Division, The Johns Hopkins Hospital, 1961.

123. Charles D. Flagle, Ira W. Gabrielson, Abraham Soriano, and Martin M. Taylor. *Analysis of Congestion in an Outpatient Clinic*. Baltimore, Md., Operations Research Division, The Johns Hopkins Hospital, 1959.

124. Milton Friedman and Simon Kuznets. *Income from Independent Professional Practice*. New York, National Bureau of Economic Research, 1945.

125. Eli Ginzberg. *A Pattern for Hospital Care*. New York, Columbia University Press, 1949.

126. W. Lee Hansen. "Shortages and Investment in Health Manpower," in *The Economics of Health and Medical Care*. Ann Arbor, Mich., Bureau of Public Health Economics and Department of Economics, The University of Michigan, 1964. Pp. 75-91.

127. John H. Hayes, ed. *Factors Affecting the Costs of Hospital Care*, Vol. 1, Financing Hospital Care in the United States. New York, Blakiston, 1954.

128. Arlene S. Holen. Effect of State Licensing Arrangements in Five Professions on Interstate Labor Mobility and Resource Allocations. M.A. Thesis, Columbia University, New York, 1962.

129. Arthur W. Jones and Francisca K. Thomas. *Report of the Hospital Survey for New York*. Vol. 3. New York, United Hospital Fund, 1938.

130. Herbert E. Klarman. "Requirements for Physicians," *American Economic Review, Papers and Proceedings,* 41: No. 2 (May, 1951), 633-45.

131. Herbert E. Klarman. "The Economics of Hospital Service," *Harvard Business Review*, 29: No. 5 (September, 1951), 71-89.

132. Herbert E. Klarman. "The Increased Cost of Hospital Care," in *The Economics of Health and Medical Care*. Ann Arbor, Mich., Bureau of Public Health Economics and Department of Economics, The University of Michigan, 1964. Pp. 227-54.

133. Eric Klinger and Helen Hoffer Gee. "The Study of Applicants, 1958-59," *Journal of Medical Education*, 35: No. 2 (February, 1960), 120-30.

134. Roger I. Lee and Lewis Webster Jones. *The Fundamentals of Good Medical Care*. Chicago, University of Chicago Press, 1933.

135. Paul A. Lembcke. "Hospital Efficiency—A Lesson from Sweden," *Hospitals*, 33: No. 7 (April 1, 1959), 34-38, 92.

136. Maurice Leven. *The Income of Physicians*. Chicago, University of Chicago Press, 1932.

136. a. H. Gregg Lewis. *Unionism and Relative Wages in the United States*. Chicago, University of Chicago Press, 1963.

137. Henry D. Lytton. "Recent Productivity Trends in the Federal Government: An Exploratory Study," *Review of Economics and Statistics*, 41: No. 4 (November, 1959), 341-59.

138. John D. Millett. *Financing Higher Education in the United States*. New York, Oxford University Press, 1953.

139. National Manpower Council. *A Policy for Scientific and Professional Manpower*. New York, Columbia University Press, 1953.

140. Willard C. Rappleye. *Personnel—The Key to Effective Health Programs*. New York, Josiah Macy, Jr., Foundation, 1950.

141. Gaston V. Rimlinger and Henry B. Steele. "An Economic Interpretation of the Spatial Distribution of Physicians in the U. S.," *Southern Economic Journal*, 30: No. 1 (July, 1963), 1-12.

142. Charles G. Roswell. "Hospital Costs—Their Components, Variations, and Future Trends," in *Conference on Cost and Quality of Hospital Care in Greater New York*. New York, Foundation on Employee Health, Medical Care and Welfare, 1961.

143. Anthony J. J. Rourke, in "Can Hospital Costs be Lowered?" Debate with Eli Ginzberg. New York, Town Meeting of the Air, 1952.

144. Jerry Allen Solon. "The Public's Image and the Nursing Home's Vision," *Nursing Homes*, 11: No. 4 (April, 1962), 8-10.

145. George J. Stigler. "The Tenable Range of Functions of Local Government," in *Federal Expenditure Policy for Economic Growth and Stability*, Joint Economic Committee, 85th Congress, 1st session, 1957. Pp. 213-19.

146. Ray E. Trussell and Frank van Dyke. *Prepayment for Hospital Care in New York State*. Albany, N. Y., State Superintendent of Insurance, 1960.

147. Herman G. Weiskotten, Walter S. Wiggins, Marion E. Altenderfer, Marjorie Gooch, and Anne Tipner. "Trends in Medical Practice—An Analysis of the Distribution and Characteristics of

Medical College Graduates, 1915–1950," *Journal of Medical Education*, 35: No. 12 (December, 1960), 1071–121.

148. Grover C. Wirick, Jr. An Econometric Analysis of the Cost of Hospital Care in the Buffalo, New York, Area. Ann Arbor, Mich., Bureau of Hospital Administration, University of Michigan, 1963 manuscript).

149. David McCord Wright, ed. *The Impact of the Union*. New York, Kelley and Millman, 1956.

150. Donald E. Yett. "An Economic Study of the Hospital Labor Market," in Daniel Howland, *The Development of a Methodology for the Evaluation of Patient Care*. Washington, D.C., U. S. Public Health Service, 1960. Pp. 231–62.

D. ORGANIZATION AND PLANNING

151. Brian Abel-Smith. "Hospital Planning in Great Britain," *Hospitals*, 36: No. 9 (May 1, 1962), 30–35.

152. D. Airth and D. J. Newell. *The Demand for Hospital Beds*. Newcastle-upon-Tyne, University of Durham, King's College, 1962.

153. Odin W. Anderson. "Trends in Hospital Use and Their Public Policy Implications," in *Proceedings of the Fifth Annual Symposium on Hospital Affairs: Where Is Hospital Use Headed?*. Chicago, Graduate School of Business, University of Chicago, 1964. Pp. 2–5.

154. Norman T. J. Bailey. "Calculating the Scale of Inpatient Accommodation," in Nuffield Provincial Hospitals Trust, *Towards a Measure of Medical Care*. London, Oxford University Press, 1962. Pp. 55–65.

155. Richard M. Bailey. An Economic Analysis of Private Medical Practice Organization, D.B.A. Dissertation, Indiana University, Bloomington, Ind., 1963.

156. E. Dwight Barnett. "Hospital-Specialist Relations: A New Look at an Old Problem," *Trustee*, 8: No. 12 (December, 1955), 19–22.

157. Mark S. Blumberg. "Distinctive Patient Facilities Concept Helps Predict Bed Needs," *Modern Hospital*, 97: No. 6 (December, 1961), 75–81.

158. Agnes W. Brewster and Lucy M. Kramer. "Health Insurance and Hospital Use Related to Marital Status," *Public Health Reports*, 74: No. 8 (August, 1959), 721–36.

159. Ray E. Brown. "Let the Public Control through Planning," *Hospitals*, 33: No. 23 (December 1, 1959), 34–39, 108–9.

160. John Maurice Clark. *Guideposts in Time of Change*. New York, Harper, 1949.

161. John Maurice Clark. *Economic Institutions and Human Welfare*. New York, Knopf, 1957.

162. Commission on Hospital Care. *Hospital Care in the United States*. New York, The Commonwealth Fund, 1947.

163. a. Robert E. Coughlin and Walter Isard. *Planning Efficient Hospital Systems*, Philadelphia, Regional Science Research Institute, 1963.

  b. Robert E. Coughlin, Walter Isard, and Jerry B. Schneider. *The Activity Structure and Transportation Requirements of a Major University Hospital*. Philadelphia, Regional Science Research Institute, 1964.

164. Michael M. Davis and C. Rufus Rorem. *The Crisis in Hospital Finance*. Chicago, University of Chicago Press, 1932.

165. Paul M. Densen, Eva Balamuth, and Sam Shapiro. *Prepaid Medical Care and Hospital Utilization*. Chicago, American Hospital Association, 1958.

166. Paul M. Densen, Sam Shapiro, Ellen W. Jones, and Irving Baldinger. "Prepaid Medical Care and Hospital Utilization," *Hospitals*. 36: No. 22 (November 16, 1962), 63–68, 138.

167. Paul J. Feldstein and Jeremiah J. German. Predicting Hospital Utilization—An Evaluation of Three Approaches. Chicago, American Hospital Association and Blue Cross Association, 1964 manuscript).

168. Gordon Forsyth and Robert F. L. Logan. *The Demand for Medical Care*. London, Oxford University Press, 1960.

169. Eliot Freidson, "The Organization of Medical Practice and Patient Behavior," *American Journal of Public Health*, 51: No. 1 (January, 1961), 43–52.

170. Eli Ginzberg and Peter Rogatz. *Planning for Better Hospital Care*, New York, King's Crown Press, 1961.

171. Hospital Council of Greater New York. *The Master Plan for Hospitals and Related Facilities for New York City*. New York, The Hospital Council, 1947.

172. Herbert E. Klarman. *Background, Issues and Policies in Health Services for the Aged in New York City*. New York, Interdepartmental Health Council, 1962.

173. Herbert E. Klarman. "Effect of Prepaid Group Practice on Hospital Use," *Public Health Reports*, 78: No. 11 (November, 1963), 955–65.

174. Herbert E. Klarman. *Hospital Care in New York City*. New York, Columbia University Press, 1963.

175. Morris London and Robert M. Sigmond. "Are We Building Too Many Hospital Beds?" reprinted from *Modern Hospital*, 1961.

  a. Vol. 96, No. 1 (January), pp. 59–63.

  b. Vol. 96, No. 5 (May), pp. 95–100.

  c. Vol. 97, No. 2 (August), pp. 79–83.

176. Millard F. Long. "Efficient Use of Hospitals," in *The Economics of Health and Medical Care*. Ann Arbor, Mich., Bureau of Public Health Economics and Department Economics, The University of Michigan, 1964. Pp. 211–26.

177. Walter J. McNerney, and Study Staff. *Hospital and Medical Economics*. 2 vols., Chicago, Hospital Research and Educational Trust, 1962.

178. Osler L. Peterson. *Quantity and Quality of Medical Care and Health*. Paper delivered before section on medical sociology of American Sociological Association. Washington, D.C., August, 1962.

179. Milton I. Roemer. "Bed Supply and Hospital Utilization: A Natural Experiment," *Hospitals*, 35: No. 21 (November 1, 1961), 36–42.

180. George Rosen, "Provision of Medical Care: History, Sociology, Innovation," *Public Health Reports*, 74: No. 3 (March, 1959), 199–209.

181. Gerald D. Rosenthal. Hospital Utilization in the United States. Ph.D. Dissertation, Harvard University, Cambridge, Mass., 1962.

182. Max Shain and Milton I. Roemer. "Hospital Costs Relate to the Supply of Beds," *Modern Hospital*, 92: No. 4 (April, 1959), 71–73, 168.

183. Sam Shapiro, Louis Weiner, and Paul M. Densen. "Comparison of Prematurity and Perinatal Mortality in a General Population and in the Population of a Prepaid Group Practice, Medical Care Plan," *American Journal of Public Health*, 48: No. 2 (February, 1958), 170–87.

184. John B. Thompson, Oscar Wade Avant, and Ellawyne D. Spiker. "How Queuing Theory Works for the Hospital," *Modern Hospital*, 94: No. 3 (March, 1960), 75–78.

185. Richard M. Titmuss. *Essays on "The Welfare State."* London, George Allen and Unwin, 1958.

186. Ray E. Trussell and Frank van Dyke. *Prepayment for Medical and Dental Care in New York State*. Albany, N. Y., State Superintendent of Insurance, 1962.

187. U. S. Public Health Service. *Areawide Planning for Hospitals and Related Health Facilities*. Washington, D.C., Government Printing Office, 1961.

188. U. S. Public Health Service. *Research in Hospital Use: Progress and Problems*. Washington, D.C., Government Printing Office, 1962.

189. Josephine J. Williams, Ray E. Trussell, and Jack Elinson. *Family Medical Care under Three Types of Health Insurance*. New York, Foundation on Employee Health, Medical Care and Welfare, 1962.

E. MEASURING PRICES AND COST-BENEFIT

190. Kenneth J. Arrow. "The Measurement of Price Changes," in *The Relationship of Prices to Economic Stability and Growth*, Joint Economic Committee, 85th Congress, 2nd session, 1958. Pp. 77–87.

191. Mark S. Blumberg. "Evaluating Health Screening Procedures," *Operations Research*, 5: No. 3 (June, 1957), 351–60.

192. I. S. Blumenthal. *Research and the Ulcer Problem*. Santa Monica, Calif., The Rand Corporation, 1960.

193. Howard Lee Bost. An Analysis of Charges Incurred for Inpatient Care in General Hospitals. Ph.D. Dissertation, University of Michigan, Ann Arbor, Mich., 1955.

194. Earl E. Cheit. *Injury and Recovery in the Course of Employment*. New York, John Wiley, 1961.

195. Ronald W. Conley. The Economics of Vocational Rehabilitation. Ph.D. Dissertation, Johns Hopkins University, Baltimore, Md., 1964.

196. Frank G. Dickinson. *The Cost and Quantity of Medical Care in the United States*. Bulletin 66. Chicago, Bureau of Medical Economic Research, American Medical Association, 1948.

197. Frank G. Dickinson and Charles E. Bradley. *Comparisons of State Physician-Population Ratios for 1938 and 1949*. Bulletin 78. Chicago, Bureau of Medical Economic Research, American Medical Association, 1950.

198. Frank G. Dickinson. "What We Get for What We Spend for Medical Care," in *Financing a Health Program for America*, Vol. 4 of President's Commission on the Health Needs of the Nation, *Building America's Health*. Washington, D.C., Superintendent of Documents, 1952. Pp. 17–23.

199. Otto Eckstein. "A Survey of the Theory of Public Expenditure Criteria," in National Bureau of Economic Research, *Public Finances: Needs, Sources, and Utilization*. Princeton, N. J., Princeton University Press, 1961. Pp. 439–94.

200. Rashi Fein. *Economics of Mental Illness*. New York, Basic Books, Inc., 1958.

201. Martin S. Feldstein. "Review of Weisbrod's *Economics of Public Health*," *Economic Journal*, 73: No. 289 (March, 1963), 129–30.

202. Joseph W. Garbarino. "Price Behavior and Productivity in the Medical Market," *Industrial and Labor Relations Review*, 13: No. 1 (October, 1959), 3–15.

203. Milton Gilbert. "The Problem of Quality Change and Index Numbers," *Monthly Labor Review*, 84: No. 9 (September, 1961), 992–97.

204. Richard Goode. Comment on paper by Rashi Fein, "Health Programs and Economic Development," in *The Economics of Health and Medical Care*. Ann Arbor, Mich., Bureau of Public Health Economics and Department of Economics, The University of Michigan Press, 1964. Pp. 282–85.

205. Seymour E. Harris. *National Health Insurance and Alternative Plans for Financing Health*. New York, League for Industrial Democracy, 1953.

206. A. G. Holtmann. *Alcoholism, Public Health, and Benefit-Cost Analysis*. Paper delivered before National Institutes of Mental Health Seminar, Bethesda, Md., December 6, 1963.

207. Ethel D. Hoover. "The CPI and Problems of Quality Change," *Monthly Labor Review*, 84: No. 11 (November, 1961), 1175–85.

208. Maynard M. Hufschmidt, Chairman, Panel of Consultants to Bureau of the Budget. *Standards and Criteria for Formulating and Evaluating Federal Water Resources Developments*. Washington, D.C., Bureau of the Budget, 1961.

209. Herbert E. Klarman. *Measuring the Benefits of a Health Program—The Control of Syphilis*. Paper delivered at the Brookings Institution Conference on Public Expenditures, Washington, D.C., November 8, 1963.

210. Howard Laitin. The Economics of Cancer. Ph.D. Dissertation, Harvard University, Cambridge, Mass., 1956.

211. E. A. Langford. "Medical Care in the Consumer Price Index, 1935–56," *Monthly Labor Review*, 80: No. 9 (September, 1957), 1053–58.

212. Louis Lasagna. *The Doctors' Dilemmas*. New York, Harper, 1962.

213. D. S. Lees. "The Economics of Health Services," *Lloyds Bank Review*, New Series, No. 56 (April, 1960), 26–40.

214. Herbert E. Levine. "A Small Problem in the Analysis of Growth," *Review of Economics and Statistics*, 42: No. 2 (May, 1960), 225–28.

215. Ronald McKean. *Efficiency in Government through Systems Analysis*. New York, John Wiley, 1958.

216. Leonard W. Martin. *Limitations on the Measurement of Costs of Medical Care*. Paper delivered before the Chicago Chapter of the American Statistical Association, Chicago, Ill., November 22, 1960.

217. Robert Merrill. "Some Society-wide Research and Development Institutions," in National Bureau of Economic Research, *The Rate and Direction of Inventive Activity: Economic and Social Factors*. Princeton, N. J., Princeton University Press, 1962. Pp. 409–34.

218. Selma J. Mushkin. "Health as an Investment," *Journal of Political Economy*, 70: No. 5, Part 2 (October, 1962, Supplement), 129–57.

219. Selma J. Mushkin and Francis d'A. Collings. "Economic Costs of Disease and Injury," *Public Health Reports*, 74: No. 9 (September, 1959), 795–809.

220. Gunnar Myrdal. "Economic Aspects of Health," *Chronicle of the World Health Organization*, 6: No. 7–8 (August, 1952), 203–18.

221. D. J. Reynolds. "The Cost of Road Accidents," *Journal of the Royal Statistical Society*, 119 (1956, Part 4), 393–408.

222. Jerome Rothenberg. *Economic Evaluation of Urban Renewal: Conceptual Foundation of Benefit-Cost Analysis.* Washington, D.C., The Brookings Institution, 1963 (manuscript).

223. John M. Russell, "Medical Research: Choked by Dollars," *Harper's* Special Supplement, The Crisis in American Medicine, 221: No. 1325 (October, 1960), 153–57.

224. Barkev S. Sanders. "Discussion of Structure, Uses and Inadequacies of the Official Price Deflators," *Proceedings of the Business and Economics Statistics Section of the American Statistical Association*, Washington, D.C., The Association, 1959. Pp. 320–22.

225. Anne A. Scitovsky. "An Index of the Cost of Medical Care—A Proposed New Approach," in *The Economics of Health and Medical Care.* Ann Arbor, Mich., Bureau of Public Health Economics and Department of Economics, The University of Michigan, 1964. Pp. 128–43.

226. George J. Stigler (Chairman, Price Statistics Review Committee). *The Price Statistics of the Federal Government.* New York, National Bureau of Economic Research, 1961.

227. U. S. Veterans Administration, Department of Medicine and Surgery. *Report of the Committee on Measurement of the Quality of Medical Care.* Washington, D.C., The Administration, 1959.

228. E. A. van Steenwyck. In *Hearings on Bills Relative to a National Health Program*, Part 1, Subcommittee of the Committee on Labor and Public Welfare, U. S. Senate, 81st Congress, 1st session, May–June 1949. Pp. 405–16.

229. Burton A. Weisbrod. *Economics of Public Health.* Philadelphia, University of Pennsylvania Press, 1961.

230. Jack Wiseman. "Cost-Benefit Analysis and Health Service Policy," *Scottish Journal of Political Economy*, 10: No. 1 (February, 1963), 128–45.

INDEX

Abel-Smith, Brian, 29, 32, 138, 141, 142
"Abuse" of insurance benefits, 32, 34, 37
Abuses under workmen's compensation, 46
Adams, Ralph, 86, 87
Afford, what U. S. can, 14, 173–76; determinants of nation's expenditures, 175
Aged population, 29, 44, 53, 71, 73, 109, 138; see also Health insurance
Airth, D., 138, 139, 141, 143
American Hospital Association, 7
American Medical Association, 7, 46, 101, 128
Ancillary services in hospitals, 135–36, 155–56
Anderson, Odin, 25, 31, 32, 33, 34, 36, 66, 132, 139, 143
Area-wide planning for hospital care, 136–44; see also Planning and coordinating
Arrow, Kenneth, 3, 11, 14, 15, 21, 26, 33, 37, 38, 49, 50, 51, 52, 56, 79, 88, 95, 111, 113, 150, 160
Average cost, 106; when not calculable, 119–20, 166

Bailey, Norman, 131
Bailey, Richard, 83, 100, 129, 151, 153, 154
Bane, Frank, 86, 100, 129, 155
Barnett, Dwight, 136
Bator, Francis, 48, 49, 50, 51, 115, 122
Bauer, Peter, 52
Baumol, William, 49, 51, 120, 145, 165, 166
Bed, hospital: definition, 103; effect on use, 140–41; estimating requirements 137–39; number, 6, 103, 137; occupancy, 125; proposals on construction, 124–25

Benefits of health programs, see Costs and benefits
Benefits under health insurance, see Health insurance
Berke, Mark, 114, 115
Blank, David, 90, 95
Blue Cross plans, 36, 44, 70, 71, 119, 120, 123, 136
Blue Shield plans, 71, 136
Blumberg, Mark, 107, 142, 171
Blumenthal, I. S., 168, 169, 170, 172, 173
Board of trustees, 57, 114, 132
Bost, Howard, 38, 155, 156, 162
Boulding, Kenneth, 11, 48, 51, 54, 122, 163, 174
Brewster, Agnes, 138
British Working Party on Nurses, 161
Brown, Ray, 16, 103, 110, 119, 141, 147
Buchanan, James, 11, 49, 53, 66, 115
Burkhead, Jesse, 48, 163, 175, 176
Business as source of financing: contributions to health insurance premiums, 33, 38, 42–43, 175; expenditures for in-plant health services, 45; workmen's compensation, 45–46

Cheit, Earl, 46, 47, 166, 169
Ciocco, Antonio, 14, 79
Clark, John, 54, 97, 110, 111, 139, 145
Closed panel plans, 128
Coinsurance, 37–38
Collective good, definition, 49; examples, 52
Commission on Financing Hospital Care, 107, 155, 156
Commission on Hospital Care, 137, 142
Committee on the Costs of Medical Care, 97

Price elasticity — pp. 24-25, estimates are probably too low

are p 21

Income elast. — pp. 26 ff, p 29

Weisbrod — p. 29